STEPHANIE

One of God's Wonder Kids

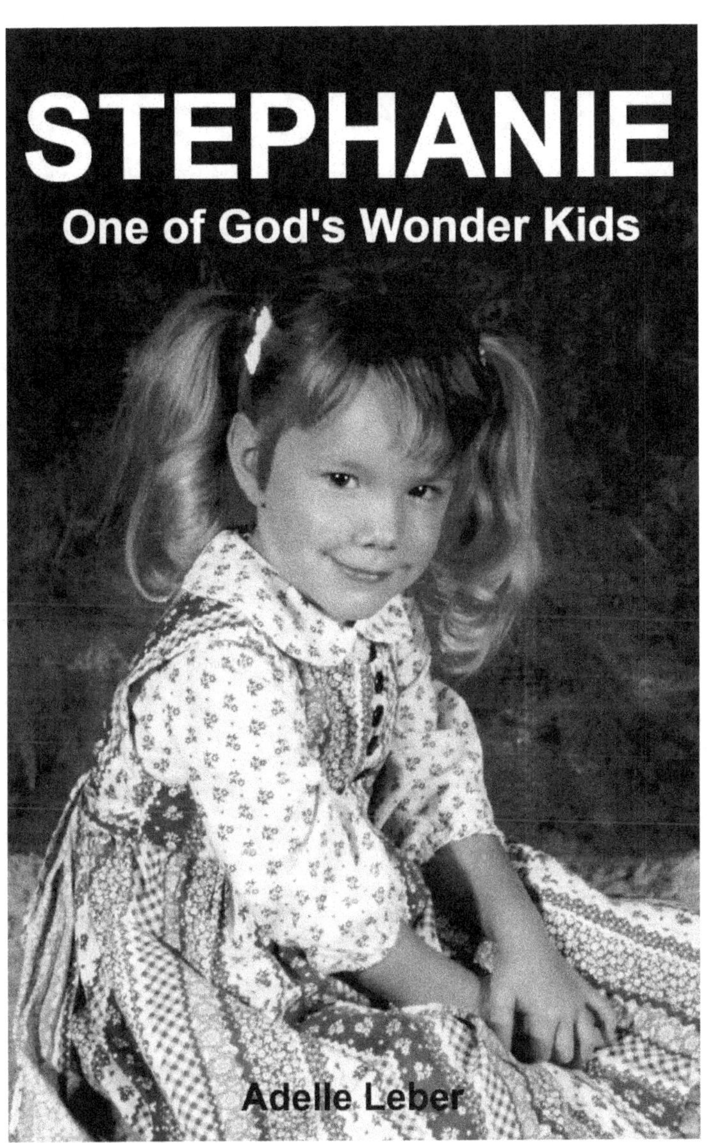

Adelle Leber

STEPHANIE:
ONE OF
GOD'S WONDER KIDS

by

Adelle Leber

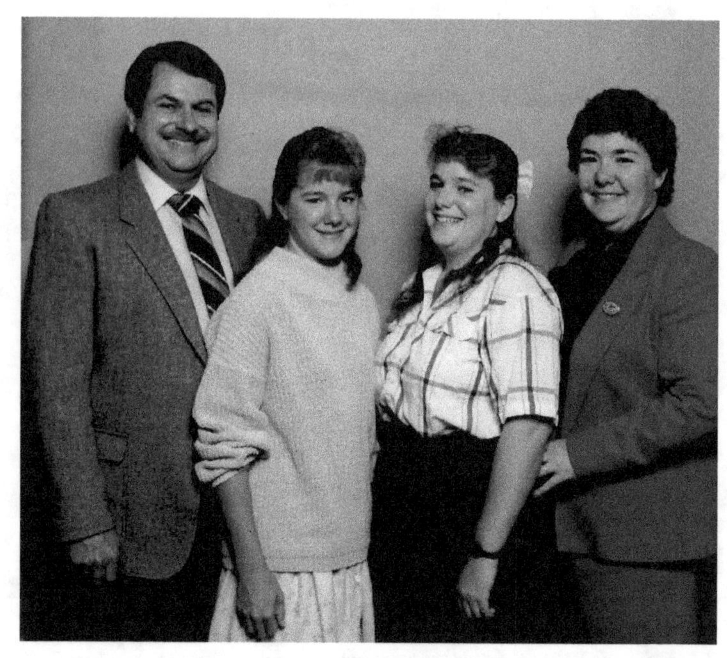

Our Last Family Portrait

Promise

John 14:27 (KJV)

Peace I leave with you, my peace I give unto you: not as the world giveth, give I unto you. Let not your heart be troubled, neither let it be afraid.

Prayer

Dear Lord,

I need inner peace and strength more now than ever before. You are the only one who can give it to me. I plead with you now: help me through this time of trouble and give me the peace and strength to face it in a calm and rational manner.

Chapter 1

Brain Tumor!

"Dr. Tomassi, our thirteen-year-old daughter, Stephanie, has had migraine headaches since she was nine years old," I said. "My husband, Steve, has had them since he was eleven years old, and so did his mother. My older daughter, Roni, also has them. Steve and Roni have had CT scans, and everything was normal. The reason I have brought Stephanie in to see you is because her migraines have become more frequent. She has started having them about once a week.

"Mrs. Leber, what are Stephanie's headaches like?"

"They are of a different type than the rest of the family. Steve's and Roni's both deal with blind spots and vision disorders, but Stephanie's seem to be more in the right side of her face and right arm. She gets numb and has difficulty moving her right side. We brought her to see you because we heard there was medication available to prevent this type of migraine."

Dr. Tomassi prescribed medication for Stephanie.

Then I said, "Steve works across the street at Loma Linda University Medical Center as chief technologist of neuroradiology. Should Stephanie have a CT scan? Steve said he could work her in for a CT scan if you wanted one."

The doctor said he usually would not order a CT scan because of the family history, and this appeared to be a "textbook" case. However, since Steve worked there, and they had time to scan her, we could go ahead with the scan.

I took Stephanie straight over to the medical center. They were just finishing with their last patient and started Stephanie right away. After she was positioned in the scanner, Steve and I went to another room to look up the medication and find out what the possible side effects might be.

While we were looking up the medication, the tech came in and said, "Steve, I think you better come have a look at this. Adelle had better wait in your office."

Steve and I both knew right then that something was wrong. While I was still waiting for Steve to come back, the doctor in charge of the CT lab came in to have me sign the consent form to use "contrast." I really knew then that something was wrong. The contrast is used to highlight an area that is suspicious.

Steve came back while she was explaining to me some of the side effects of the contrast. He took the consent form, said, "I know them all. Go ahead," and signed the paper. Then he told me that they'd found a tumor in the middle of her brain.

We just stood there and cried.

When they finished the CT scan, they said they needed to do a Magnetic Resonance Image (MRI) because it would give them more detail of the tumor and the area. A CT scan uses x-rays to develop a slice or image on a TV screen whereas an MRI is developed from magnetic waves and displayed on a TV screen.

Two hours later, we were in the MRI waiting room. While all this was going on, the neuroradiology doctors were deciding which one of them would be the best for this particular case. They unanimously decided it should be Dr. David Knierim, a leading neurosurgeon.

As soon as the MRI scan was finished, Dr. Knierim was there "reading" the scan, and he talked to us right away. He said the tumor was about the size of a walnut and was positioned in or near her thalamus. He could not tell for sure exactly how involved it was. He suggested surgery but gave us virtually no hope for a long-term survival. The tumor had sealed off the normal drainage of the ventricles in her brain and was causing increased pressure. He stated that having to go surgically through the center of her brain would most likely cause other complications, some of which might be paralysis, diabetes, blindness, thyroid problems, or death. If we did nothing, that would result in certain death very soon.

This was October 20, 1987. We went ahead with plans for surgery despite all the possible side effects. It would be November 5, 1987.

Promise

Psalm 55:22 (Living Bible)

Give your burdens to the Lord. He will carry them. He will not permit the godly to slip or fall.

Prayer

Dear Lord,

You have to carry my burdens and me through this time. I cannot survive without You and still keep my sanity.

Chapter 2

Initial Reactions of Family and Friends

That first day, October 20, was a day I would not want to live through again. Even sitting here writing this is extremely difficult.

Since then, people have asked me, "What was the very first thing that entered your mind when they told you that Stephanie had a tumor?"

I must be honest, the very first thing I thought of was that God has promised that we will never have to go through more than what we can endure, with His help.[1] I decided right then and there that God must have felt we were able to endure this or it would not be happening. If God felt that way, who was I to disagree? Therefore, we would survive. If it was to God's glory that Stephanie die, so be it. I cried, I hurt, but I knew "this too shall pass." God has also promised that all things work

---

[1] Phil. 4:13.

together for good to those that love the Lord.[2] Furthermore, I believe that when we do get to heaven and are going over all the events that have happened, and we can see from the beginning to the end, we shall see how He used everything to His glory, and we will say, "God, I wouldn't change a thing. I would go through it all again."[3]

It was hard to tell Stephanie that she had a tumor. But she took it very calmly. Basically, she reacted the same way I did: "Okay, what happens next? What will it do to me? What will I go through? What if we do nothing? What is the worst I can expect?" She didn't break down and cry until Dr. Knierim started explaining what would happen during surgery. They would start by *shaving her head!* They lost her right there. That affected her more than anything else.

Take a moment and think about a thirteen-year-old girl losing her hair. That is when girls really start becoming interested in boys. They start worrying about how they look. To have *no hair...* That crushed her. She really had no problem with anything else the doctor had explained to her— just the *no hair*. We went out the next week and let her pick out a wig, which eased her feelings a little.

Steve talked to Stephie the next day about losing her hair. She said she couldn't imagine what she would look like with no hair. Steve remembered the woman in *Star Trek: The*

---

[2] Rom. 8:28.

[3] Ellen G. White, *Prophets and Kings* (Nampa, ID: Pacific Press, 2002), 578).

Motion Picture who had a bald head. He got the video and showed it to her. She saw how pretty that woman was and accepted the fact, and she said she could live with *no hair*.

Steve had a harder time accepting Stephanie's condition than I did. He very seldom showed it on the outside, but he was crushed inside. Continuing to work at Loma Linda University Medical Center in the neuro-angio department was really hard for him because every day he had to look at the scans of other people with tumors and know that his daughter had one too! Steve had always felt for other families, knowing what they would be going through, but never expected to see his own family in that same situation. He also hurt for the other families, knowing what they were going through and still had to face.

The night of October 20, Steve had to drive down to San Pasqual Academy (a coeducational Christian boarding school) to tell our older daughter, Roni, what was happening. We also decided that it would be best if she came back to live at home again and be near the family, especially Stephie. We also knew Roni would take this news hard and would not survive emotionally away from home at a boarding school. Steve had to go by himself so they would have room for all of Roni's clothes and belongings. We had called beforehand and talked to the dean so that she would know what was happening but asked her not to tell Roni. Steve wanted to do that himself. By the time Steve got there, the dean had already set up a place where Steve and Roni could be alone. The dean had also gotten several people together who would help pack and load all of Roni's things. There was a lot of hugging and crying.

How Stephie Affected Me

By Roni

When I first heard about Stephanie, I was on my way to PE class. I saw my dad driving up the driveway to the girl's dorm and wondered why he was here. When he saw me, he stopped the car and said we had to talk. I told him I'd be free after PE class, but he said *no*, we had to talk now.

After he parked the car, he looked me straight in the eyes and said, "Stephanie has a brain tumor."

I said, "No, she just has headaches like you and me."

He repeated it again, "No, she has a brain tumor!"

That time, we both started crying and hugging each other. Then he asked me if there was a place we could go and talk. I told him I'd have to go and tell Mrs. Brandmeyer that I was not going to PE, but he said he'd called before driving down and everyone knew what was happening. We went into the girls' dorm to use one of the side rooms.

Mrs. Brandmeyer came out and asked me if I was all right and gave me a big hug. It was then that Dad told be how they'd found out Steph had a tumor, how Steph was dealing with it, and kind of what to expect in the future. I asked him how quickly it was growing, and he said he didn't know, but the doctor said she might live up to a year and half. We both started crying again and hugged each other and prayed together. We asked Jesus to give us all strength to get through this as a whole family.

When we walked out of the room, Mrs. Davis, my work supervisor, was waiting to talk to me. She gave me a big hug, and we started crying again. I told her that my sister had a brain tumor, and we both cried even harder and just stood there hugging each other. Mrs. Brandmeyer had arranged for a couple of my friends to help pack all my belongings so that I could go home.

One of my friends came up to me and hugged me and handed me a piece of paper with some Bible texts on it and said, "These always give me strength when I need it the most."

They all helped load the car. Dad had to sign some paperwork taking me out of school, and we left.

On the way home, we listened to a music album by the Goads and cried the whole way. The thing I remember most about the ride home was that it was the longest ride from school I had ever been on. When we got home, Steph came out to help unload.

She saw us crying and said, "Please don't cry. I don't want you to be unhappy."

I will never forget that because it told me right there that she was the most caring person and that she really had Jesus in her heart.

How Stephanie affected her school

Fairview Junior Academy

On October 21, Steve and I went to Stephanie's school, Fairview Junior Academy (a Christian day school), to talk to the principal and take her out of school. The principal was out of town, but his assistant, Mr. Rice, one of Stephanie's teachers, was there. We told him that she had a brain tumor and we had been given virtually no hope. The three of us sat there and cried. Finally, we calmed down enough to get back to reality and tried to figure out what to do next. We said that, basically, we couldn't plan the future until after surgery and we had received the results.

Fairview Junior Academy had just started their week of prayer. Believe me, that was a week the students will not forget. A local minister, Pastor Dave Bottroff, was the speaker that week. He really got a workout. The students and teachers came to him for counseling on how to deal with this tragedy. "Pastor Dave" came to see us and to talk to Stephanie and see if he or anyone else could do anything to help us. Just knowing he was there was a big help. Throughout this ordeal, he was one of our mainstays.

The teachers at Fairview Junior Academy got together to come up with something the students could do to help

Stephanie. On November 3, we found out what they had planned as a surprise for Stephanie. She was scheduled to be admitted into the hospital on the fourth for an "angio." During an angio, a small plastic tube or catheter is introduced into the femoral artery in the groin and is advanced to different areas of the body to visualize the vascular system. In Stephanie's case, they wanted to see which vessels of the brain were supplying blood to the tumor.

The catheter is positioned using a fluoroscope with x-rays. When it is in position, a high-contrast fluid that shows up on x-rays is injected, displacing the blood, which can't be seen. The x-ray film then displays a road map of the blood vessels involved near the injection. After the angio, Stephanie was to spend the night at the hospital and have surgery on the morning of the fifth.

The school had arranged with the hospital's public relations personnel to have Stephanie put in a room next to the window so that she'd be able to see the parking lot after her angio. Four school buses drove into the lot with all the students from the school. They put large banners on top of the buses that said, "We love you," "God loves you," and "Get well soon." They also had a big banner that the lower grades had made with all their signatures. The hospital had arranged for four walkie-talkies—three in the parking lot with the kids and one up in Stephanie's room—and they let all the kids talk to Stephanie. When they were about to leave, they all let balloons go with prayers inside. We can never thank the school enough for having gone to all that trouble for us. It really boosted all our spirits. I think it helped the rest of us as much as Steph—maybe even more.

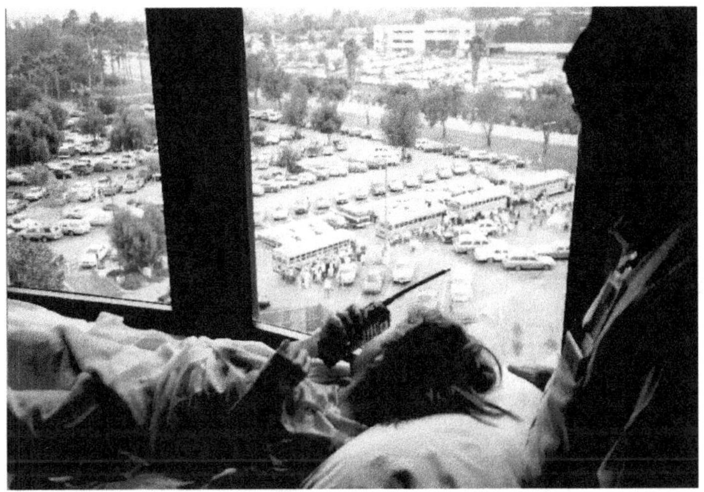

After that, I think everybody in the hospital knew who Steph was. They couldn't believe that someone could be loved so much. That was also when we started to realize just how large an impact our little girl had made and was still making on other people's lives. We knew she was a sweet, well-liked girl, but we never realized how much. The school told us later that they were originally going to bring only the eighth graders over, but when the rest of the school found out, everyone wanted to come. They said they all loved her and wanted her to know that. Around 160 students and teachers became involved.

That evening, we had Pastor Lenart and the elders from our church come to anoint Stephanie.[4] Satan was really

---

[4] See James 5:14.

working that night. The young girl in the bed next to Steph's was on a respirator that made horrendous noise, she had an IV (intravenous injection system), and she was hooked up to every possible monitor. During the anointing, all her alarm bells went off. The respirator went off, the IV bell went off, and her heart monitor buzzer started going. All of this was going on during our prayer circle, but we didn't let this stop us. We continued to pray and ask the Lord for a special healing, for guidance of the doctor's hands, and for a peace upon all of us who had to just sit and wait.

Jesus Wept

By Dad

As a boy growing up, I cried for various reasons without thought of the fact that others saw me. Then around ten years old, I realized that if I wanted to show others I was becoming a man, I couldn't allow others, including my peers, to see my weakness by crying or even letting tears form. Suppressing those strong emotions was tough, but I worked at it until I did a pretty good job of it.

One occasion that I remember was when I was around the age of twelve. We were living in Costa Mesa, CA. The county was putting in a six-foot cement storm-drain pipe on the corner by our house. The crane involved needed to swing into our yard to place the pipe. We needed to remove the top three layers of cement blocks from our wall on the street side to allow this. We were able to salvage the bricks and found that striking the edge of them with a hammer caused the old mortar to drop away. It took a solid tap for this to happen, and after doing a few, I felt pretty cocky at having mastered it so quickly. What increased the feeling was my mother and younger brother watching me.

Well, as is often the case in a situation like this, my concentration relaxed, and my thumb got in the way of one of the solid taps. They both saw it happen. The pain didn't hit right away. It started slowly as a throbbing and finished with the most excruciating pain I had ever felt. It didn't split the skin, but a blood blister formed under the nail, causing the throbbing pain.

Now the point of the story: I didn't cry. There were some tears but no crying. My brother made me proud when he said, "Mom, Steve didn't cry or anything."

When a time comes in our lives when we feel that crying would destroy our "manly" or "macho" exteriors or that crying would cause us to lose face in front of others, then a little bit of ourselves has died.

When we discovered Stephanie's tumor, the shock of the moment, along with trying to deny the whole thing, prevented the tears and crying from coming out. Soon, however, I wanted to cry but couldn't let that emotion surface. Holding back those tears took a lot of willpower. I loved Steph, which made it that much harder to do, especially when so many around me were very emotional.

Adelle had stayed with Steph all night at the hospital. At seven in the morning, I was backing out of the drive to go in and see how she had done through the night and to relieve Adelle so she could have some breakfast. I turned on the radio and thought maybe some oldies but goodies might lift my spirits. Listening to religious music was very difficult for me because it made me want to break down and cry. The very first song that played was "Bridge over Troubled Water" by

Simon and Garfunkel. That was all I could stand. I had to release all my pent-up emotions I had kept inside.

I quickly pulled off to the side of the road and cried. I prayed for strength and asked the Lord to help me understand what was happening. I realized for the first time that, for a man, showing emotion does not suggest he is weak. It shows love and caring. It shows you are alive and have needs.

Jesus wept over Jerusalem in Luke 19:41. Was that a sign of weakness? Not in any sense of the word. He cared about his people and what was going to happen to them.

A large burden of stress was released that morning. Until then, I could sit through *The Sound of Music, Love Story*, etc. without a tear. I can't do that now. Not feeling the burden of having to be macho and super strong helped me to feel compassion for others, to consider their needs and feelings. It's been hard for me to accept a Christian hug from a brother in faith. Now, I understand it's a great way to let someone know you care and want to help.

Promise

Psalms 27:5, 6 (KJV)

For in the time of trouble he shall hide me in his pavilion: in the secret of his tabernacle shall he hide me; he shall set me up upon a rock. And now shall mine head be lifted up above mine enemies round about me: therefore will offer in his tabernacle sacrifices of joy; I will sing, yea, I will sing praises unto the Lord.

Prayer

Dear Lord,

I realize that this is part of my "time of trouble." I need you to set me up upon your rock and lift my head above this enemy, cancer and death. I want to sing your praises, but I don't have the strength. Please give me the stamina to keep going.

Chapter 3

Surgery and Results

Stephanie's preparation for surgery started about six in the morning on November 5, 1987. The medical team had already done the lab work but had to do some more. We were allowed to stay with her for a lot of the prepping. Then they took her away. That was hard.

Because Steve worked at the hospital, we were allowed to use the x-ray techs' lunch room as our waiting room. That was a good thing, for we filled the room with our friends. A few friends were with us the whole waiting period, and several others couldn't stay the whole time but came and went. Sometimes, we would talk and other times we just sat there, each of us thinking individual thoughts. We talked about a lot of different subjects. We got to know each other better during this time. A few of our friends didn't know each other even though they knew us, so we talked about each other's history and background. We also talked about God and how He had led us so far, how good He had been to us. We talked about how we didn't know why this was happening but that we knew God was in control and everything would work out to His glory.

One of our friends had made lunch and put it in the lunchroom refrigerator so that all we had to do was heat it up. Knowing a lot of people would be there, she had made enough casserole to feed all of us. That was very nice. Even though we weren't really hungry, we knew we had to eat.

We have a lot of friends who are nurses, and they were able to go into the operating room and bring us progress reports. Finally, about four in the afternoon, they reported that she was through surgery and was being taken to the recovery room.

They informed us that she had come through the surgery wonderfully. She was already recognizing people and moving all her limbs, so we knew she was not blind, deaf, or paralyzed. To us, that in itself was a miracle. Dr. Knierim had told us that damage would "very likely" be done during surgery.

Finally, were allowed to see her, and we were very relieved to see that she'd made it through surgery okay and to give her hugs.

Stephanie had taken her favorite teddy bear, Jason, with her. The nurses were wonderful about that. They even took Jason to the recovery room so that she could hold him. They bandaged his head just like hers and gave him a baby-sized hospital gown and a hospital name band.

Because she was still heavily drugged, we went home and had a good night's sleep and praised God that Stephanie had made it through surgery so perfectly.

The next morning, my father, John Squier, went to see Stephanie very early. When he got there, Stephanie was sitting up and feeding herself breakfast. She got up and walked to the restroom to brush her teeth. I arrived a little later, and she was sitting up in the chair. By then, she was extremely tired but happy, feeling no ill effects from surgery. She had no deficits from having had her brain handled. She had no paralysis, and nothing seemed wrong with her. Nothing that we feared might happen had happened. We were all praising God. We could see God's answer to our prayers in that He had definitely guided Dr. Knierim's hands. I stayed with her all day even though she slept most of the time. I sat there and held her hand. It was a miracle. Since she was doing so well, my father decided to go back home to Oxnard.

That evening, we went home for dinner. As we were walking back into the hospital, we were stopped by friends who had gone to see Stephanie. While we were talking to them, the resident on duty, Dr. Abu-Assal, came up to Steve and asked him to come into Stephanie's room. She had become unresponsive suddenly, and they were hoping that Steve's voice would bring her back to consciousness. It did not.

Dr. Abu-Assal ordered an IV be started immediately with Mannitol, a very strong diuretic, and had Steve arrange for an emergency CT scan. Steve made a call to the CT area and found the scanner was empty at the moment and told them to get it ready for Stephanie. All of this was accomplished in five minutes. The nurses couldn't believe how quickly Steve arranged for the CT until they found out that it was Steve's department. Steve and I wheeled Stephanie to the CT rooms, not having to wait for the hospital dispatch. We had her back in her room with copies of the scan within twenty minutes.

Dr. Abu-Assal sent us to the waiting room while he and Dr. Brian Craig worked on Stephanie. They performed an emergency burr-hole incision (her second surgery) so that her spinal fluid could drain out of her head. They also put her on a respirator. This was at about half past seven in the evening. They worked on Stephanie, trying to bring her to a conscious level until midnight, when she finally roused from her coma.

We realized again how really seriously ill Stephanie was. Knowing something and really realizing it are two different things. We could also see how Satan was trying to discourage us and get us to turn away from God. We knew God was in control, and if Stephanie was to die, it would be to God's glory, not Satan's.

During all of this, Steve and I were devastated to have our hopes raised so high and have them dashed again. We called Pastor Dave, and he came to be with us "on the double." He spent the whole night with us, talking to us and praying with us. That night was one of the hardest for me. It was even harder than when they'd first told us she had the tumor. I still didn't give up hope, and I still believed that God would give us the strength to make it through this ordeal, but it was difficult.

What had happened is called post-surgery swelling. The brain swelled because it had been disturbed. It had been swelling ever since the surgery, but it took that long to reach the point where no more room existed inside the skull to swell. The skull, being bone, can't stretch like skin can when swelling occurs in another part of the body. When the brain is under pressure, it starts to shut down. That's what we call going into a coma or unconsciousness. Therefore, the reason they inserted the catheter and gave her the diuretic was to eliminate as much fluid as possible as quickly as possible. And, of course, the purpose of opening the burr hole and inserting the drainage channel directly into the brain ventricle was to eliminate as much pressure on the brain as quickly as possible. The respirator was also used to help eliminate moisture. For some reason, the respirator is beneficial in solving the problem as well.

The next morning, when I was able to see Stephanie, that was very traumatic for me. Walking in and seeing my thirteen-year-old "baby" with a bandage on her head and a tube sticking out, hooked up to a container on the wall with clear reddish fluid in it, an IV in her arm, a catheter coming out the end of her bed to a bag hanging on the side, and a noisy respirator with tubes in her mouth was almost too much for me. I'm sure it was a result of God's providential care that she was asleep and couldn't see my face when I first saw her.

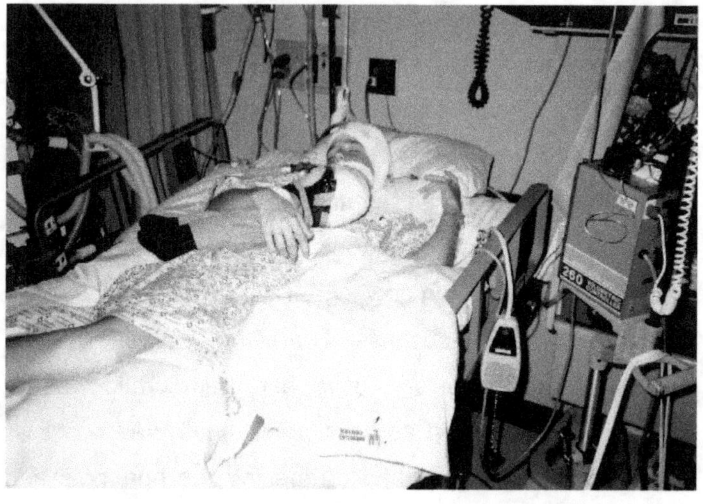

I sat down and held her hand until she woke up. That's when we discovered she was totally paralyzed on her right side. The pressure on the brain had done some damage. Stephanie wasn't aware she was paralyzed. Whenever they asked her to move, she thought she was moving. She couldn't raise her head because of all the tubes, so she couldn't see what was or was not happening. After the third day, they finally held up her hand so she could see it and asked her to move her right fingers. Her eyes got huge when she saw that they were not moving. Then she got this strained look on her face, and we knew she was doing everything in her power to move her fingers. From then on, about every half hour, I held her hand up for her to see, and she would try to move.

When the doctors realized she was paralyzed, they told us that she probably wouldn't come out of it. They wanted to tell Stephanie that, and I said, "No! You will never tell her anything is hopeless. When you are in front of her, I want you always to be as positive as possible." The doctor said the staff would go along with my wishes.

After a week of paralysis, a couple of her fingers started to move. The Lord had renewed her strength and power and determination to move.

Stephanie was on the respirator for a week. Her right lung had also been affected, so she had to stay on the respirator until her lungs were strong enough to function on their own. While Stephane was on the respirator, her sister, Roni, would come every day and rub body lotion on her arms and legs. Roni even shaved her legs one day. Even though Stephanie couldn't talk, you could tell by her face what she needed and enjoyed.

Stephanie's school friends were wonderful. Many of them came to see her as often as the nurses would allow. Even with all her tubes and everything, they would come and just hold her hand. Seeing young people being so caring was very refreshing. Also, several of Stephanie's nurses were parents of her friends. That's why a lot of rules were bent in order for them to see her at odd hours. We had told the whole staff that if they felt Stephanie was up to it, anyone could see her, but if they felt she was too tired, they should send them away. We felt that the visits would help keep her spirits up and let her know how many people cared. The nurses told me they had never had a patient with so many friends that would come to visit. Staff also came to visit her. They were impressed and happy for her.

When they finally did remove the respirator, we discovered Stephanie couldn't talk in her normal voice. All she could do was whisper. Dr. Knierim ordered the speech specialist to come and check her out. He found that the tube they had used for the respirator was too large and had done some damage, and half of her vocal cords were still paralyzed as well. He said her voice should come back but not quite to normal. Steph's voice did become louder than a whisper. She could not yell or talk very loudly, but really, who cares?

Once Stephanie started to improve, she did so at a miraculous rate. Dr. Knierim couldn't believe how quickly she started getting her strength back. On November 12, 1987, Stephanie went into surgery again (her third surgery), but everything was okay that time. They were putting an internal shunt in so that she could get rid of the tube coming out of her head. They removed the respirator on November 13, 1987.

On Saturday, November 14, 1987, Stephanie was the recipient of a very special treat. Six young men, a Christian singing group called The Master's Plan, gathered around her bed in the hospital and sang six inspirational songs. Totally acapella, this very good group would go around to the local churches and sing. One of the members is our neighbor, and he and his group wanted to do something for Stephanie. They didn't go around to sing to anyone else, but many others, patients and staff, came to Stephanie's room.

The nurses just couldn't get over how much attention and love Stephanie received. She had gotten so many flowers and stuffed animals and cards that the nurses had to find an extra table for her. We also had to take some home because the hospital room just wasn't big enough.

The doctor sent her home on November 19, 1987 after only two weeks in the hospital. Dr. Knierim had told us before the surgery that she would be in the hospital at least two months. He saw how we took care of her and knew we would be able to take care of her at home. We had a very happy Thanksgiving because our "baby" was home. She was on a lot of medication but was doing great.

Promise

2 Corinthians 7:4 (Living Bible)

I have the highest confidence in you, and my pride in you is great.
You have greatly encouraged me; you have made me so happy in
spite of all my suffering.

Prayer

Dear Lord,

Thank you for being there when we need you the most. Thank you
for carrying my burdens. Thank you for encouraging others to do
things that lighten our load. Thank you.

Chapter 4

Hawaii, a Happy Interlude

The social worker at the hospital helped us get in touch with a support group, the Starlight Children's Foundation. It is a foundation, supported only by donations, that grants last wishes to terminally ill children. They arranged for our whole family, all four of us, to go to Hawaii, and they paid for everything. They had arranged for four nights at the hotel, but we wanted to stay the week, so we said we would pay the difference. When we arrived at the Surfrider Hotel, we asked how much we owed for the additional nights, but they said it would be taken care of and we shouldn't worry but have a good time.

We arrived in Honolulu on December 4, 1987, to a stretch limo waiting to take us to the hotel. When Starlight was arranging this trip and asked Stephanie what she would like, she told them she wanted to ride in a limo. So that is what they arranged. Her face just beamed when the driver was standing there with our name, and he led us down to the limo, took care of all our luggage, and stood there holding the door open for Stephanie. She couldn't believe she was riding in a limo. She knew nobody could see in, but we had fun watching them try to see which celebrity was driving by. That was a big thrill for her.

The hotel assigned us to a suite on the twentieth floor. We had two balconies. One was right over Waikiki Beach with a view of Diamond Head.

One early morning, Stephanie and I were sitting on the balcony, and she was looking out across the water. She didn't like to look straight down because we were on the twentieth floor, and sometimes she would get a little dizzy. But this morning, she was looking at the water and spotted some dark movement. We went inside and got binoculars and then could see the shapes were large sea turtles. From then on, we watched the turtles. They would come out early in the morning looking for food then go away when people got in the water. Stephanie was proud that she saw them first.

On our first afternoon, we rented a car and drove around the island till the road ended, then we came back. On the way back, we stopped at a beach that had beautiful sand. We had worn our swimming suits just in case, so we walked down to get wet and have fun. I didn't realize that the beach quickly sloped down. I didn't want to be in water that deep, so I turned around to walk back to shore, but a huge wave hit me, lifted me in the air, and plopped me hard on my tailbone. Stephanie was the first to get me to help. Roni and Steve were laughing too hard. They all had to help me get back to the car, I was hurting so badly. I didn't have much fun, but everyone else enjoyed that beach.

The hotel's public-relations director had arranged for a special outing for us every day. She arranged one thing per day, and the rest of the time was ours. We didn't know what Stephanie would be able to do, and we didn't want to overtire her.

One day, we went to the Polynesian Cultural Center. I think this day was Stephanie's favorite because there was so much to see and we were treated like royalty. The PR director had arranged for a wheelchair, so all we had to do was go to the ticket window and say who we were, and they had everything ready for us. Every place we went, they put Steph right up front so she could see. We didn't have to go through lines because wheelchairs went in a different area, where those guests could see better.

Each of the different Polynesian islands had its own area to show what their history and culture was like. Steph liked the Tonga area because she got to try swinging the poi balls. She thought that was great fun. In fact, we had to buy her some so she could keep practicing. But her favorite was the Tahitian dancing. We even got a video of her trying the Tahitian dance.

I need to explain here that when we found out that we were going to Hawaii, an unknown donor rented a video camera for us. We still don't know who did that, but we are so thankful.

We were told to take all the pictures of her that we could because they would be important later.

Another day, we went to the Sea Life Park. Again a wheelchair was waiting for us, but this was one of Steph's better days, so she would get out and push it, using it like a walker. Steph enjoyed watching the dolphin show and watching the sharks swim around. Steph's favorite area was the turtle pool. We got to ask about the turtles we were watching at Waikiki Beach. The staff confirmed that they were snapping turtles and that they stayed away from people.

At one point, Roni was pushing Steph around, and Steve and I were walking ahead. Apparently, Roni was not going fast enough for Steph because we turned around just in time to get a video of Steph pushing Roni down a slight decline at a run. Roni's face showed pure terror, but Steph was beaming. It was just luck that we happened to get it on video. That is special to us.

Another morning, we went to Waimea Falls. Steph's favorite things there were not the foliage, trees, and birds, but the "buff" cliff divers. We went up and met them afterward. That was the highlight for Steph. We also got some pictures of Steph and Roni in a canoe. One fellow there was playing a ukulele and singing some Hawaiian tunes. He was singing a bit off-key, to the point that even Steph was cringing a little bit and wondering how long he was going to continue, but it was still fun.

One of the mornings, we went to Hanauma Bay, where people can snorkel. If you want the fish to come up to you there, you feed them frozen peas. Trust me when I say you want them to come to you. The fish are amazing.

That evening, we went to the Sheraton's Polynesian Review, a dinner and dance show. We got to see a luau, where we got to have traditional Hawaiian food, and the dancing was amazing. We had a great time that night.

One day, we just drove around the island and enjoyed all the different beaches, stopping off at the Byodo-in Temple and Pearl Harbor. Steph enjoyed the Byodo-in Temple, where she got to ring a big bell by pulling back a big log with a rope and letting it go. Then the log hit the big bell, making a very pleasant gong. Her favorite moment there was working with the caretaker of the temple. He would whistle, and birds would come and eat out of our hands or off our heads or shoulders. Steph thought that was great.

We had a glorious time, relaxing and enjoying ourselves as a family. We returned home on December 10, 1987.

Promise

Isaiah 25:4 (RSV)

For thou hast been a stronghold to the poor, a stronghold to the needy in his distress, a shelter from the storm and a shade from the heat; for the blast of the ruthless is like a storm against a wall.

Prayer

Dear Lord,

Again, I feel the urgent need for your strong, loving hands to reach down and take my inner soul into your shelter from the storm.

Chapter 5

Radiation Treatments

By the time we returned, the doctors had all the reports from pathology and oncology, and the tumor board had come to their conclusions on how to treat her tumor. The tumor board is a group of specialists that come together to discuss difficult cases. They informed us that the surgery she'd had was really nothing more than a biopsy because the tumor was totally involved in the thalamus. All that Dr. Knierim had been able to do was take the center out of the tumor. Therefore, what was left would have to be treated with radiation. The tumor board had concluded that proton acceleration, which is being used for some tumor treatments at Berkley, CA, would not be beneficial in Stephanie's case. They also felt that chemotherapy's side effects wouldn't be offset by the benefits. They thought that the best and only course of action would be to use radiation.

On December 17, 1987, radiation treatments started. The schedule they set up was twice a day, five days a week, for seventy-three treatments. The treatments needed to be at least four hours apart, so we had to drive to the hospital's oncology department twice a day. Her appointments were at 7:30 a.m. and noon.

Dr. Catalano did allow Stephanie to have a one-week break from the radiation treatment so the she could go to Camp Ronald McDonald for Good Times. This is a very special camp for kids with cancer. Camp Ronald McDonald was even equipped to handle the kids who are on chemotherapy. The camp has staff there that can give any treatment necessary. We were impressed with their love and dedication to the campers. They have a staff of fifty-five and only allow one hundred campers at a time.

Stephanie was really excited about going until we arrived at a meeting point outside the camp and saw all these kids, some with no hair, some with partial hair, and some very sick because they had just received a chemotherapy treatment. I think when she saw how sick some of these kids were, it finally dawned on her how sick she was. Stephanie said she didn't want to go to camp after all, and she cried when she got on the bus to go on to the camp. Making her go and seeing her crying like that was really hard for me. As they were pulling out, I saw one of the staff come and sit with her and hug her.

When they came back at the end of the week, Stephanie was all smiles. She'd had a wonderful time. The camp was great, and the staff really know how to treat these kids. They play lots of games and also have talk sessions in small groups. The kids talk out their anger about "Why me!" and tell each other what all they have had to go through. They discuss how "normal" kids have treated them because the campers either have no hair or scraggly hair. The camp helped Stephanie realize that people had to accept her the way she was, with no hair, and that her appearance was not her fault.

Stephanie finally finished the radiation treatments on February 10, 1988. She was very lucky that she had minimal effects from the radiation. Most people become ill and sick to their stomachs, but Stephanie had only a short time of being tired. We looked at this as another blessing from God.

They radiated the tumor from three directions. That way, no one spot on her head received too much radiation. Stephanie did lose her hair on both sides of her head, in circles just over each ear. Those were the points of radiation. The other point was on her forehead, so she had no hair loss there. Dr. Catalano, who was in charge of her oncology treatments, informed us that she might not get her hair back in those two spots, but again Stephanie was blessed, for it did grow back.

Promise

Romans 8:28 (KJV)

And we know that all things work together for good to them that love God, to them who are the called according to His purpose.

Prayer

Dear Lord,

Thank you for your guidance and direction in our lives. Thank you for preparing the way to make this time of trouble a little easier for us. Thank you for being there and loving us.

Chapter 6

God's Providential Guidance

You know, in looking back, I can see how God guided our lives to prepare us for this tragic event. If it had happened three years earlier, I would have been out of a job. At that time, I was working for a certified public accountant. Leroy Luyster wouldn't have been able, even though in his heart he would have wanted, to let me off during November, December, January, February, March, and April. Those are his busiest months of the year, tax time. I hadn't been looking for a job when I left the CPA's office. A friend called me and offered me a job at a convalescent hospital. At that time, I felt God was leading me, and I accepted her offer. God knew what I would need three years in the future though I surely didn't.

In March of 1986, I decided that I really wanted to complete my college education, get my BS degree, and become an administrator of a convalescent hospital. I enrolled in the Whitehead Program at University of Redlands. It is an accelerated program in which one can earn two years of units in one year. I finished the program in March of 1987, but graduation was in June.

After class completion, I was asked when I wanted to start the Administrator-in-Training (AIT) program. The still small voice inside me said to wait, back off, relax. I made my decision in August 1987, to put the idea of AIT in limbo for a while. Two months later, Steph was diagnosed with the tumor. If I had been in the middle of the AIT program, I wouldn't have been able to stay home. These might seem like coincidences to some people, but I really believe God was opening and closing doors.

Steve also believes God was leading in his life, preparing him also. He was baptized as a Seventh-day Adventist in February 1974, a month before Stephanie was born. When Stephanie was about two months old, Steve was lying on the couch one Saturday afternoon, and all of a sudden, he sat up and said, "Did you hear that?"

I said, "What? I didn't hear anything."

He said, "I just heard God speak to me. He told me I should quit my job and go back to school full time at Loma Linda University, La Sierra Campus. What do you think?"

I told him to check it out. Then we discussed all the realities, financially etc., everything "fell into place." He was accepted by the university. My parents had a house in La Sierra that we could live in if we just paid the property taxes. With the funding available to Steve through the VA education program, we could make it. Then Steve had to decide what he wanted to take. The Lord led him to choose x-ray technology. While Steve was still going through the x-ray courses, he found he really liked neuroradiology, so he specialized in that. Receiving a degree in x-ray technology entails one year of basic courses on the La Sierra campus and two years on the Loma Linda campus. After these two years, another year is spent in specializing. While Steve was in his year of specialization, he was hired by Loma Linda University Medical Center as a technologist. Steve eventually worked up to become chief technician of the neuroradiology department.

Just think—if Steve had not been in that position, we would not have had a scan done and found the tumor as early as we did. Also, because he was the chief tech, he had the freedom to come to visit Stephanie several times a day while she was in the hospital. There again, we believe God was in control.

During all this, I felt I was being run ragged. I had to take Stephanie to see Dr. Knierim and Dr. Catalano and to get follow-up CT scans and MRI scans and radiation treatments. I felt as though I was never home. I am very thankful that we lived only three miles from the hospital and the doctors' offices. I was also trying to work at my regular employment during all this. I must add here that I was very thankful for my employers, who allowed a lot of adjustments in the office at Crestview Convalescent Hospital, where I was office manager. They allowed me to bring a computer terminal home and hook it up to the main computer through a modem and phone line, to work at home. In order for things to work smoothly, we had to adjust many of the job assignments. Some things I did could be done at home, and some couldn't be done out of the building, so everyone cooperated by letting me do their work that could be done out of the building, and they took over mine that couldn't.

Steve had this to say about his career change during that time:

> I had been with the medical center for almost ten years. At first, it seemed wonderful because of the freedom it gave me to visit Stephanie. Also, knowing many of the doctors and department heads allowed for an easier time scheduling the different treatments and doctor visits she required. However, knowing as many people as I did soon started affecting me. As I would pass friends and acquaintances in the hall, they all wanted to know how Stephanie was doing. After several months, I didn't want to leave my office because of all the encounters it meant in getting to my destination. They were caring and loving people, but they didn't see that the same questions were being asked me over and over all day long. In January 1988, I heard of a sales position with Fuji Medical Systems, selling x-ray film and equipment. I applied for the position and was hired in April. That still allowed me the freedom to be home if needed or to help out with appointments for Stephanie.

Promise

Philippians 4:4 (KJV)

Rejoice in the Lord always: and again I say, Rejoice.

Prayer

Dear Lord,

I know we are to rejoice always no matter what happens. That is not easy. We do not feel like rejoicing during this hard time, facing the death of our daughter. But we know we are to rejoice, so we rejoice that You are there going through this with us.

Chapter 7

Continuing Impact and Adjustments

When the radiation was completed, we thought, *Well, that's it. All we can do now is sit back and wait to see what happens.* This thought gave me a mixed feeling. It's nice to say, "Okay, I have done all I can, and it is now in God's hands." But not knowing what to plan for or what to expect is also frustrating. Waiting for an uncertainty is not easy.

During this time, we arranged for a home tutor through the Colton Joint Unified School District's special-education program. That's a program set up for children who physically cannot attend school. Her teacher, Mr. Gene Edelbrock, came to the house every afternoon for about one to two hours. We did this to give Stephanie as normal a life as possible. We wanted to give to her the hope that when she improved, she would be able to carry on normally, go back to school with her friends, and still be in the same class with them.

She still spent a lot of time with her friends. They would come and hang out. They would share different stories about what was happening at school. These stories would help stuff. She would laugh and enjoy them.

I know it had to be hard for her friends seeing Steph like that. I do know that each of them loved Steph and Steph loved them. I know that Joy, Laura, and Renaldo will always have a special place in Steph's heart.

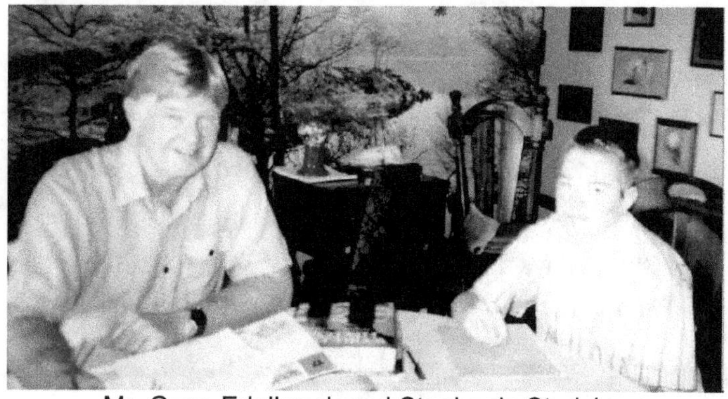

Mr. Gene Edelbrock and Stephanie Studying

Promise

Philippians 4:7-8 (Living Bible)

If you do this, you will experience God's peace, which is far more wonderful than the human mind can understand. His peace will keep your thoughts and your hearts quiet and at rest as you trust in Christ Jesus.

And now, brothers, as I close this letter, let me say this one more thing: fix your thoughts on what is true and good and right. Think about things that are pure and lovely, and dwell on the fine, good things in others. Think about all you can praise God for and be glad about.

Prayer

Dear Lord,

We are at another low. These verses tell us to keep looking for the positive, but right now, I do not see any. You have to trigger my memories. I cannot overcome my agony. You have to pull me up again.

Chapter 8

Relapse: Tumor Growing Again

On February 11, 1988, Stephanie was not feeling quite normal. She said her right arm felt "funny." I noticed that she was losing some coordination. She tried to scratch her nose and hit her forehead. She started using her left hand more and more. She would get up from the TV to go to her bedroom and walk into the wall. By February 15, 1988, she was starting to drag her right leg. It did not seem to want to cooperate. She was becoming lethargic and very listless. Her right arm would fly out of control, and she would have to sit on it or hold it with her left hand. Her speech became more difficult. This was a hard time for all of us. Seeing your daughter deteriorate right before your eyes is not easy.

The family had already decided that we did not want her to go back to the hospital if that were at all possible to avoid. Steve talked to Dr. Knierim, and he ordered an MRI scan. That was scheduled for February 17, 1988 at seven in the evening, but Stephanie woke up that morning with an extreme headache and vomiting. When Steve got to work, he talked to the doctors, and they said to bring her immediately for a CT scan. He called me, and Stephanie and I were there in ten minutes. This CT scan showed that the tumor had grown since December. It had been about the size of a walnut, but now it was the size of a small tangerine. Dr. Knierim came and looked at the scans and said we had a choice between doing nothing or letting him put in two more shunts. That would not help much with the tumor, but it would give us a few more days. The tumor had grown around the shunt and was keeping it from draining. With the amount of pressure that had built up in her brain, she would probably only live a few days.

We decided that since nothing more could be done to remove the tumor, because it was so entwined with her thalamus, it was not worth the trauma of her going through surgery again only to give her a few more days. She would be in a hospital with a lot of tubes again and not at home where we could really hold her and love her. We brought her home and arranged for hospice to help with anything we were not able to do. Hospice is an organization more concerned with the quality of remaining life than with prolonging life. Hospice stresses controlling pain and maximizing the patient's comfort. It is also concerned with the needs of the family members as well as those of the patient.

Promise

Philippians 4:19 (KJV)

But my God shall supply all your need according to his riches in glory by Christ Jesus.

Prayer

Dear Lord,

You are obviously filling Stephanie's needs. She is so calm and accepting. She is a strength to us. Thank you.

Chapter 9

Stephanie's Faith and Trust in God

That afternoon, we told Stephanie exactly how serious her condition was at the moment. She knew her condition was not good, but she hadn't realized that she was getting that close to dying. However, learning that she was dying didn't seem to upset her. She took it very calmly.

The "grapevine" works very well. That afternoon and evening, we had a lot of visitors. Pastor Lenart and Pastor Dave just happened to arrive at the same time. Stephanie had gone into her bedroom to lie down just before they arrived, so they both went in to talk to her. They both came out shaking their heads. They could not believe they had just been talking to a thirteen-year-old. They told us we didn't have to worry about Stephanie. She understood she was dying and was ready. What was upsetting her was not that she was dying but how much we would miss her and how much we would be hurting.

She was not angry or scared. She knew that dying would be like going to sleep and then waking up to see Jesus' face smiling down at her.[5] When the pastors told us that, Steve and I both had tears rolling down our cheeks.

Stephanie walked out about that time and saw us crying, and she grabbed Kleenex, wiped our eyes, and said, "It's okay. I'm ready."

Stephanie was a special gal. She knew what she wanted to be when she grew up. When she was nine years old, she had to have her teeth straightened. When she saw what kind of car the orthodontist drove, she decided that was the job for her. She thought it would be neat to help people look better, and of course the money wouldn't hurt. She never gave up on that dream.

Stephanie always had lots of friends. She was a good leader. She was not afraid to step out and volunteer to do anything, but she always had enough sense to realize whether or not it was something she could do. She wouldn't do something if it was dangerous or stupid.

Stephanie and her friends would get together and have lots of fun, but she knew what was right and what was wrong as far as the Lord in her life.

Stephanie was a good student in school. She enjoyed school. She very seldom had a problem unless it was math, which was not a good subject for her.

---

[5] I Thess. 4:14-17.

I think the best description of what Stephanie was like was given at her funeral by Mr. Rice, one of her teachers. The following is a transcript of his speech:

One of my first memories of Stephanie was really more of a nightmare than anything else, not because of Stephanie but because it was on good old bus number 7. From second to fifth grade, I was Stephanie's bus driver.

I remember very clearly it was the first week of school—a busload of students I didn't really know and a long hot trip home. I expected trouble from the big bad junior-high boys, not from two little blond girls in the second grade—that was Misty and Stephanie. These little girls could talk endlessly and loudly.

When we started the route, they were sitting across the aisle from each other up in the front by me. As the route went on and the bus emptied, the girls decided that it would be fun to move to the back of the bus. At first, I didn't really notice. But one seat at a time, these two little girls, who were in dresses and looked very sweet and cute, climbed over, under and around the bus seats as they worked their way to the back. The farther back they got, the louder they got.

Well, when it was time for them to get off, I went to the back and did my best to be mean and vicious and scare these little girls into behaving. I thought it worked, but her older sister, Roni, assured me, "Oh no, Mr. Rice, these two girls are uncontrollable when they get together. There is nothing you can do. There is no hope." Well, I went and circled their names on the seating chart. I knew I had to remember these girls.

Well, I don't honestly remember another incident on the bus or in the classroom where Stephanie was anything but courteous and respectful. She was never really any trouble again. And in her class, that was truly a feat. Trouble had so many different names and faces.

Stephanie was a good student. She cared about her classwork. She wanted it to be on time. She wanted it to be right. She tried hard to do this in all of her classes. She was a doer, not a watcher. She cared about people. She was involved. She participated in school activities, the play days, the banquets, the parties, etc. She was in Junior High Choir with Mr. Morgan.

She stayed for intramurals, one of just a handful of girls who would stay for after-school sports—football, mind you. I still remember her and Tina, two of my littlest, tiniest girls, playing football with the boys. They both showed so much courage and tenacity in pulling those boys flags. I still remember helping to teach her to throw a football on the sidelines during a game.

"Not like a girl, Mr. Rice," she said. "I want to throw a spiral."

And it took some work and some time, but she did it. And you've never seen a bigger smile than when she had mastered throwing a spiral.

Life at Fairview is supposed to be a conservative Christian environment. I don't think anyone was a better example of that than Stephanie. During this whole experience, the courage she showed left people dumbfounded. It was unbelievable. The hundreds of lives and hearts that were touched can never be measured. She was proof while she was with us, and she will be everlasting proof when Jesus comes again, that when you love Jesus and have faith in Him and believe His promises, you will be saved. She knew and believed this.

I refuse to be sad today because she would say, "Mr. Rice, stop it, you know better." Because she will be whole and healthy when she opens her eyes and sees Jesus's face. We can't survive in this sin-filled world or expect to have eternal life except through Jesus.

Stephanie and her life should serve as a constant reminder to all of us of what our purpose is here and what we can accomplish when Jesus is the head of our team. A dedicated Christian family—Steve, Adelle, and Roni— you provided the foundation and the environment needed. You gave her your all, everything she needed. The Rialto Church, the pastor, the leaders, the Pathfinders, her friends, etc. all provided the vital aspects of her Christian growth. The school, of which I was proud to be a part—we were there to try to teach her more than math and science. She is proof and will be through all eternity that we can survive and succeed in this world.

I know of no greater joy that anyone could ever experience than to know we helped a child along their way to heaven. We can rejoice today. We have succeeded.

Promise

Psalms 84:11 (KJV)

For the Lord God is a sun and shield. The Lord will give grace and glory: no good thing will he withhold from them that walk uprightly.

Prayer

Dear Lord,

Thank you for your protection and for sending such wonderful friends to help comfort and support us. Every little thing helps. Thank you.

Chapter 10

Continuing Support from Friends

I had scheduled Stephanie to get a manicure and a pedicure that day when Steve called and said to bring her in for the emergency CT scan, so I had to cancel. When we got home, I called Molly, the lady that was going to do the manicure, and asked her if she could come to the house and give her one anyway. She said that she didn't drive but if someone could come get her, she would love to. I went to get her about seven that evening. I had told her all that had happened that day, so she was prepared for a house full of people and not happy ones at that. She was wonderful with Stephanie. She and I both had to hold Stephanie's hand still so she could do the manicure. The hardest part was holding it still long enough for the fingernail polish to dry.

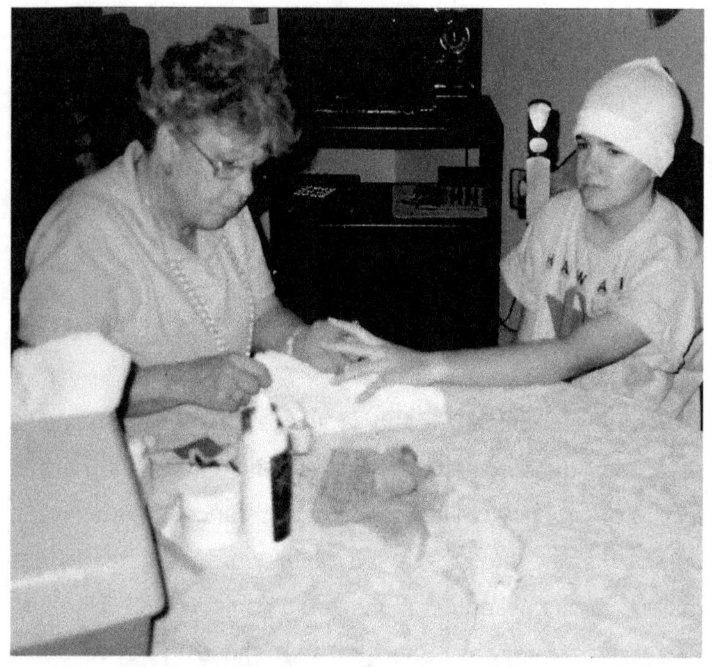

So many people had come to be sure we were okay that we ended up having a party. It really was a very nice evening. My sister, LaVon Nolan, took Molly home for me. On the way, Molly suggested that we have an early birthday party for Stephanie. That was February 17, and her birthday is March 10. LaVon called me when she got home to see how I felt about the idea. I thought about it and called her the next day. I decided I didn't want to call it a birthday party, but we would just have a big open house.

On February 21, 1988, LaVon and a neighbor of mine, Anita Strahan, hosted an open house at our house for Stephanie. Anita, Roni, and LaVon had called as many of Stephanie's friends as they could think of. They had told them to call anyone else they thought would like to come. Steve announced at church that we were having an open house and that everyone was invited. It lasted from four to eight in the evening. We could not believe how many people came to our house. In those four hours, we had over forty kids in our house the whole time, as well as between fifty and eighty adults that came and went. We hadn't told Stephanie they were coming, and she was elated.

Her friends were terrific. Somehow, they organized themselves and went in groups of three or four to sit around Stephanie and talk to her and then switch groups. My sister had rented a bottle of helium to blow up balloons, and the kids found that if they breathed it, they would talk funny. They had a lot of fun playing with that for a while. Then we got out the game Pictionary and divided everyone into two big groups. We all had a good time.

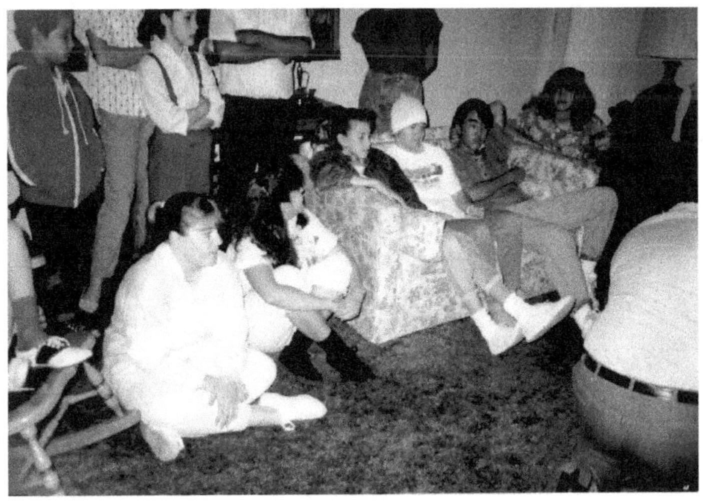

We were all very tired but happy. We had decided that we didn't want anyone to remember Stephanie in a morbid, sad way. We wanted them, and us, to remember her as a happy girl. She didn't want people to be sad. She was assured that the first thing she would know would be Jesus's face, and what is sad about that?

Stephanie kept holding her own. She would have good days and bad days as her coordination seemed to be getting slowly worse.

It was during this time, we started thinking about and planning her funeral. We bought the cemetery plot, picked out the casket, and talked to the funeral-parlor people. We also decided who would do what for the funeral. We also felt it would be nice to have the Pathfinders be the pallbearers.

Pathfinders is a coeducational youth group run by our church—similar to Boy Scouts/Girl Scouts—and Steve and I were the directors of the Rialto Pathfinder Club. Our assistant directors, Joe and Anita Mendoza, talked to the kids about being pallbearers. At first, they were upset that we were planning the funeral when she was not even dead yet. But Anita explained to them that just because we were planning it didn't mean we wanted it to happen. When they realized that we had to plan just in case, they said they would be proud to help.

Promise

Matthew 11:28-30 (KJV)

Come unto me, all ye that labour and are heavy laden, and I will give you rest. Take my yoke upon you and learn of me; for I am meek and lowly in heart: and ye shall find rest unto your souls. For my yoke is easy, and my burden is light.

Prayer

Dear Lord,

We come to you with our burden. We are claiming your promise to give us rest. Thank you.

Chapter 11

Relapse Again:
Cyst, Not Tumor This Time

We saw Dr. Knierim on March 15, 1988. We told him about all Stephanie's headaches, and he could see her loss of control of her right side, so he ordered another MRI scan just to see what was going on. The MRI was performed on March 17. My untrained eye told me it looked bigger. That night, she was not feeling very good. I helped her go to bed just after seven because she was very tired. She didn't look good to me. Her eyes were kind of glazed over and red. Her face looked puffier than usual, and she also said her eyes were blurring.

Dr. Knierim called on March 18, at about half past two in the afternoon and said he had just looked at the MRI scan again and that he didn't think the tumor had grown but that what we all saw was a cyst. The tumor was producing fluid and was filling a sac around itself. He felt it was advantageous to go in and repair the shunt and drain the cyst.

We talked it over with Stephanie. We told her that the tumor had not grown after all, that Dr. Knierim thought that if we drained the cyst, she would start improving again. We told her it was her decision if she wanted to have her head shaved again and go through all the pain and discomfort. We prayed about it, and all decided to go ahead with the surgery. We admitted her into the hospital about half past nine that evening.

On March 19, 1988, they finally took Stephanie to surgery about five in the afternoon. LaVon, John, and their son Patrick came to see us, and as soon as Stephanie was taken to surgery, they took us out to dinner. Stephanie's surgery was over about seven, and she went to recovery. Dr. Knierim came out and talked to us and said the surgery had gone very well—in fact, better than expected. They removed about thirty cc's of fluid. He also said that if the tumor didn't change, he thought we could have Stephanie with us for up to a year. As long as the shunts kept working and the tumor didn't grow, there would be no problem. He let us go in and wait with her in recovery.

Dr. Knierim saw her on the twentieth and said she was doing great. He took her off the heart monitor and took out her IV. Stephanie thought she was ready to come home. We were allowed to bring her home on March 23, 1988.

Promise

Proverbs 17:22 (Living Bible)

A cheerful heart does good like medicine,

but a broken spirit makes one sick.

Prayer

Dear Lord,

Please help us keep our spirits up. It is not easy to stay optimistic when death seems so near. But we know it is important, especially for Stephanie.

Chapter 12

Stephanie Lives as Normally as Possible

Fairvew Junior Academy said Stephanie could come to school anytime she felt well enough. Stephanie wanted to try to go to school on April 4, 1989. She lasted about half a day before she got a bad headache, but she was happy. She got to see all her friends in a normal situation again. She went to school whenever she felt well enough, clear through to June. She would go for part of a day and be home for a couple of days.

On May 8, 1988, we did another CT scan. She'd had a "horrendous" headache for four days that nothing would get rid of. She was also vomiting and had kept nothing down. We were worried that maybe the shunts had stopped working. The CT was "beautiful." The shunts were working very well. Her blood condition was normal. Thus, we guessed she just had a strange flu with a headache and vomiting but no fever. Grandma Squier gave me an old home remedy for upset stomach. She said to give her two teaspoons of concentrated

Coca-Cola syrup and, after fifteen minutes, give her one teaspoon of frozen concentrated orange juice. Every fifteen minutes, we were to give one then the other until she started feeling better. Giving her small concentrated doses wouldn't upset her stomach as much. We started the routine, and she did improve.

June 9, 1988 was a great day. Stephanie's teachers worked with her, which allowed her to graduate from eighth grade with her class. Stephanie volunteered me to play the piano. You ought to try that sometime—play *Pomp and Circumstance* on the piano when you are crying so much you can't see because your terminally ill child is walking down the aisle months after she was not supposed to live through the night. I made a few mistakes, but nobody cared. One of Stephanie's friends, Laura Boynton, gave a speech in tribute to Stephanie. There wasn't a dry eye in the auditorium. It was so moving and wonderful.

Stephanie continued about the same all summer. She had good days and bad days. She was slowly having more good days. Therefore, when school started in September, she wanted to try to attend as a full-time student. She managed only about two days in two weeks. I decided that was not fair to her, to the school, or to the other students. That was when I arranged for the home tutor again.

On October 19, 1988, we did another MRI scan. They gave her a special contrast (gadolinium-DTPA) during the MRI scan, which would highlight any part of the tumor that was actively growing. Guess what! God had performed a miracle. No live tissue was in the tumor. The doctors did not say the tumor was dead, but they would not say it was growing. We rejoiced and felt Stephanie was healed.

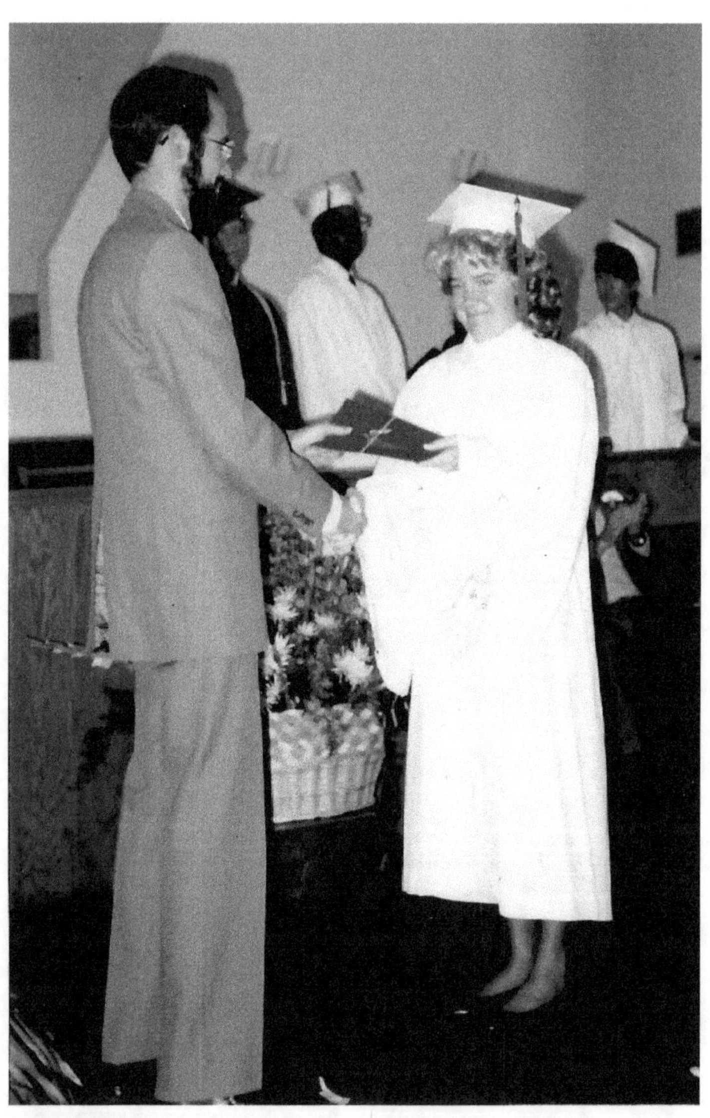

Promise

Romans 8:38 (Living Bible)

For I am convinced that nothing can ever separate us from his love. Death can't, and life can't. The angels won't, and all the powers of hell itself cannot keep God's love away.

Prayer

Dear Lord,

I am so glad that nothing can separate us, for I need You more now than ever before. I do not know why Stephanie has had to go through all this, and I may never know until I get to heaven. Only you can make my heart willing to accept this.

Chapter 13

Another Relapse:
The Emotional Roller Coaster

Three months later, on January 21, 1989, Stephanie woke up at three thirty in the morning with a "horrendous" headache and vomiting. I just thought, *Oh great, now she has the flu!* The next day, a Sunday afternoon, Stephanie started complaining that her right side felt "weird," not numb or tingling, but "weird." By Monday afternoon, she started to have deficits on her right side. She started dragging her right leg and holding her right arm a little limp, and the right side of her face was drooping a little.

I called Dr. Knierim's office and made an appointment for Tuesday, his first available appointment. He checked her and said that something was definitely going on and ordered a regular series of skull x-rays and some lab work then ordered another MRI for that night at eight. With Steve's influence, we were allowed to watch the scan being done, and as soon as it popped up on the screen, we all knew the news was not good. One of her ventricles was very enlarged again, and when they gave her the contrast (gadolinium-DTPA), the tumor "lit up like a light bulb." Dr. Knierim came in while the scan was still going on, and we started discussing our options right there.

After scheduling another shunt surgery for Thursday morning, we admitted her into the hospital on Wednesday night. Dr. Knierim called us at home about ten that evening and told us Stephanie was going to go into surgery about seven thirty in the morning, and if we wanted to see her before she went in, we should have to be there by six thirty. So we went in early to give her hugs and support.

After they took Stephanie into surgery, Steve went home to get some work done, and I went to the seventh-floor day room to wait. While I was waiting, several friends came to visit, including Donella Munson; Anita Strahan; my sister, LaVon Nolan; and Pastor Dave Bottroff.

Dr. Knierim called the day room about nine thirty and said the surgery had gone great and Stephanie was in recovery. They finally wheeled her out of recovery and to her room about noon. We got to go in and see her about twelve fifteen. She really didn't know we were there because she was so sleepy, so we left to go get lunch. When we returned at about two, she was still very sleepy, so Steve went home again, and I stayed and sat there and held her hand.

We were all more depressed this time, which we'd never thought possible. We all thought she had been healed. That whole past year and three months had been an emotional roller-coaster ride. When the doctors had first told us she had cancer, we were down. After surgery, she was doing so well that we were up. Then she went into the coma, and we were way down. Then we had a slow climb up as she kept improving until February, when she slowly started down again. Then we had an extreme high in March after that surgery. Then in October, when they told us the tumor had no live tissue, we were even higher yet. Now that they had told us her tumor came back to life and was even bigger than it had been to begin with, we were at an even lower low.

I know in my mind that God knows what is going on and will use it to His glory, but my heart was saying, "What the hell is going on? How much more are we going to be expected to endure? How is this major setback going to glorify God? How are we going to tell everybody now that God didn't do this miracle of healing like we thought? What will this do to all the people we thought we were witnessing to?" I am so glad that my faith in God was not based on my feelings, or I would have had none at that point.

Dr. Knierim came in to see Stephanie Friday evening and told us that he would probably allow her to go home Monday. Stephanie was ready to go home right then, but of course he said no. Saturday morning at nine, Dr. Knierim came in again and had Stephanie hold her arms out with her eyes closed to see if they drifted or not, and he had her get up and walk. He looked at me and asked me if it would bother me to change a dressing. I said that no, I could handle that.

Then he looked at Stephanie and said, "You can go home."

The nurse and I both looked at him and said, "Are you serious?"

Nobody had seen anybody released off the neuro floor that soon after neurosurgery. We were home by nine forty-five.

On February 15, 1989, Dr. Catalano called, and I could tell by his voice that he didn't want to be making this call. He said the tumor board had met and all agreed that nothing more could be done for Stephanie. Any more radiation would do more harm to her brain, and if they tried again to remove the tumor surgically, that would definitely cause damage. She would be paralyzed and probably in a permanent coma. He said that anything they could come up with would be just a "Band-Aid" treatment. I told him that we would follow Stephanie's wishes and would let her die peacefully at home with the help of the hospice program again. Even though we had prepared ourselves for this news, it was still very difficult to take. When we hung up, I sat there and had a good cry.

Being positive in front of Stephanie all the time was really hard. And I did feel that was important. I think the cry was good for me.

Promise

2 Thessalonians 3:16 (Living Bible)

May the Lord of peace himself give you his peace no matter what happens. The Lord be with you all.

Prayer

Dear Lord,

Thank you for all our wonderful supportive friends. You have used them to help us achieve an inner peace. We plead for your continued support to sustain that peace.

Chapter 14

Loving, Caring Friends Provide Wonderful Support

We have had support from so many friends and relatives. I know some families don't have supportive friends, family, or even a church to rely on. I really feel sorry for them and wish I could do something. We have received emotional and financial support from people we never would have dreamed of. One of our neighbors gave me a meal ticket for twenty dollars to the hospital cafeteria. That was a wonderful gift that I would never have thought of. It was a great help to me while Stephanie was in the hospital.

Financially, we were able to do quite well. Insurance covered the expense of this whole ordeal. Our out-of-pocket expenditures were small compared to the total bill, but we had a lot of hidden expenses. One major item nobody paid for was my time off work. Even though I was allowed to work at home, I was not able to work forty-hour weeks. The reason I was home was to take care of Stephanie, and that had priority.

Emotionally, my neighbors and friends and family will do anything they can if I just ask them. The problem is that when someone is in a tragic situation, they do not know what they need. They can't think clearly. All they know is that they want help, but they don't know what. Everybody reacts differently and needs different help, but all I can do is tell you what helped me the most. I loved it when people came to visit even if we didn't say anything but just sat and watched TV together, just so I was not alone.

Other times, I needed to talk. Even though I had told the same person twenty times what had happened or was happening, I needed to say it again. Sometimes, I just didn't remember if I had told that person the latest or not. Because we had as many people supporting us as we did, I couldn't remember whom I had told what.

I had trouble planning and cooking meals. I was too emotionally drained to do that even after Stephanie was home and I was home all day. I didn't mind straightening my house but didn't have the stamina for real cleaning.

I didn't mind doing laundry. We had one friend offer to do my laundry, but for some reason, I didn't want to give that up, I don't know why—unless that was just one thing that kept me in touch with normalcy. I realize everyone is different, and for some people, baking or cooking might be their emotional outlet. I guess laundry was mine.

When you hear of a person who has cancer or any serious illness, don't let your fear and emotions stop you from reaching out to that person. No matter how inadequate you feel, if you are sincere, anything will help. Just knowing you care and are praying is helpful. It doesn't really matter what you say. What is most important is that you are a good listener.

In our case, we had a lot of people praying for Stephanie. Our church family at the Rialto Seventh-day Adventist Church was a major source of support. They all prayed for us, hugged us, and loved us. Another major group was the Azure Hills Seventh-day Adventist Church. In their church service, they have what they call A Garden of Prayer. Pastor Dave Bottroff presented Stephanie's case to the church, and they started praying for her. They have ridden this emotional roller coaster with us.

One night, in particular, Steve and I both really felt at peace. We literally felt that a weight had been lifted. We found later that on that night, the members of the Azure Hills Seventh-day Adventist church had arranged for a twenty-four-hour, around-the-clock prayer session. You will never be able to convince Steve and me that prayer does not work. We felt God's peace come over us.

Some friends didn't understand me when I said I was not really praying for total healing although that would have been nice, but that my major prayer was for peace, understanding, and acceptance. I wanted to be willing to allow God to use the situation in whatever manner would glorify Him most.

If you are in a situation to help someone going through a death or an illness, you need to reach out as soon as possible with a phone call or a card, or have flowers sent or something just to let your friends know that you know they are hurting and that you care. Then offer to help in the day-to-day chores, shopping, cleaning, laundry, or cooking, or taking care of other children. To me, the most important way our friends helped us was just being available to talk. They didn't wait for me to call, they would just come over anytime. You know, God sent them to us at just the right times. Whenever our spirits were down, someone would come to the door to check up on us and to pray with us. God always knew when to send them.

According to the book *When Your Friend Gets Cancer*, by Amy Harwell, there are seven simple suggestions of what you can do.

1. Check your attitudes about cancer and about friendship. Do you secretly think of cancer as punishment? Does it sound an immediate death knell in your mind? Then you need to clarify your thinking because the cancer patient doesn't need people who will judge her and work through their attitudes in front of her. Also, think about the meaning of your friendship.

2. Reach out immediately and boldly. The cancer patient is experiencing isolation. She needs your phone call or card now.

3. Get prepped on cancer facts, figures, and feelings. Do some homework to understand basic cancer jargon and the emotional impact of the disease, especially as related to your friend's specific case. She might not have the energy to educate you herself.

4. Offer your helping hands. Lift up the cancer patient, encourage her, make her environment more pleasant, do practical nuts-and-bolts chores, support her loved ones, and steer her to other available resources. You have something special to give her that only you can provide.

5. Share your healing heart. Listen to the cancer patient. Ask her gently probing questions as she goes through her process of adjustments, especially as she deals with her changing expectations for the future. Embrace her. She needs your physical touch of love. Pray for her.

6. Help your friend make death and dying decisions (if asked). Your friend will face major decisions if her prognosis is poor. Help her as she deals with health-care ethics, as she explores her relationship with God, and as she deals with her pending death.

7. Be there for your friend. Once she has been diagnosed with cancer, her life will never be the

same. Hang in there with her as she lives with the post-treatment blues and faces a new future.

Your visits mean so much. You are showing God's love just by taking the time to say hi. You can show peace, joy, hope, and love and never have to say anything. Just your presence shows you care.

When you are being a supporter, do not be surprised if the patient or family get angry. And most of all, do not be surprised if some of it is eventually directed at you and God.

Most importantly, touch the patient and family. A person who is ill or is hurting has an increased need to be held and loved.

Prayer is an absolute must. It is a gift everyone can give, and it costs nothing. When people told me they were praying for us, that meant so much.

The longer an ordeal like ours continues, it gives you, as friends, a chance to show your true friendship by not abandoning the ones affected. It means so much for you to keep sending cards, flowers, and making the phone calls.

A word of caution: if you are helping, be sure to take care of yourself. Do only what you are comfortable doing. Do not get caught up in the events and let yourself get down. Keep yourself plugged into God and keep your energy up. Remember, God can use other people also. Do what you do best, and let others do what they do best, and God will put it all together so that it works out best for your friend.

Another major source of comfort was just hugs and touching. It is really amazing how much a hug can relieve frustration and tension.

Try to be as normal as possible with your friends. Take them out to dinner, shopping, miniature golf, or whatever they normally like to do—chances are they still do. You might have to adapt certain activities to any physical handicaps they might have, but don't make a big production out of it. Try to be as normal as possible.

Another item we found extremely helpful was an answering machine on our phone. Instead of the usual greeting, Steve prepared a special message. He would update the message whenever anything major happened to Stephanie. Our friends knew that they could call and not be a bother but could still find out how Stephanie was doing. If we were home and felt up to talking, we did, and our friends knew that we might be there but just didn't feel like talking.

We loved and appreciated all the support from our friends, Steph and Roni's friends, and all the church family. As I said before, the whole family felt the prayers working in our hearts and souls. They really helped us through one of the worst times in our lives. There is someone that we all wanted to say thank you to, and that is God. He got this family through one of the worst times it has had to face.

Promise

Psalm 28:7 (KJV)

The Lord is my strength and my shield; my heart trusted in him, and I am helped: therefore, my heart greatly rejoiceth; and with my song will I praise him.

Prayer

Dear Lord,

Thank you for being my strength. Without you, I would be nothing. I also thank you for the different agencies that have helped us have a little recreation. We need these little excursions to keep our spirits up.

Chapter 15

Disneyland

Dolores Cornejo, a clinical social worker at Loma Linda University Medical Center, arranged for our whole family to go to Disneyland. All we had to do was go to the Guest Relations Office and pick up our complimentary passes. They also provided a wheelchair for Stephanie. We went on March 8, 1989. It was a beautiful day, nice and sunny and clear but not too hot. A lot of people were there, but it was not crowded.

We arrived at Disneyland about ten thirty in the morning. We rode everything Stephanie wanted to ride. Even though Stephanie was wheelchair bound for the most part, the first ride she wanted to go on was Space Mountain, which is, of course, the roller coaster in the dark and is very exciting.

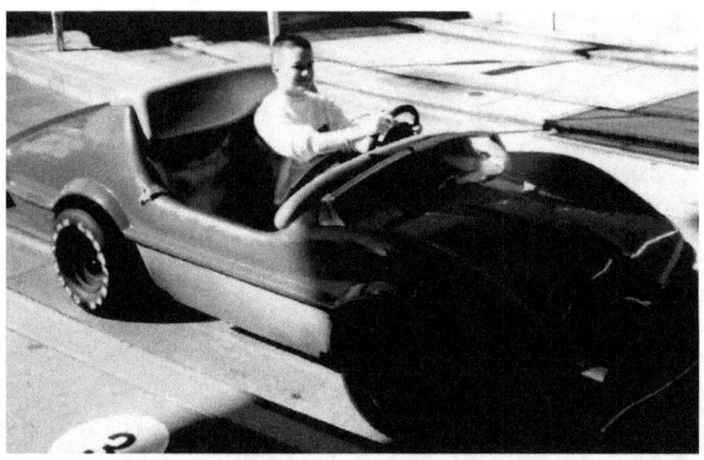

We are very thankful for the way Disneyland is set up to accommodate wheelchair visitors. When you don't have anyone in a wheelchair, it is sometimes difficult to understand why so much money goes into wheelchair accommodations. But when you have a loved one in a wheelchair, it is a blessing. The way Disneyland's workers treat wheelchair visitors is wonderful. For instance, at Space Mountain, we didn't have to try to get a wheelchair up the escalator and wait in long lines. They allowed us to go in through the exit and go down an employee hallway that put us right where they load the roller-coaster cars. As soon as we walked out with Stephanie in the wheelchair, an employee came over, helped us into a car, and held it up to make sure we were in because Stephanie walked very slowly and stepping up, over, and in was hard for her. At the end of the ride, they were right there, ready to help her out with her wheelchair ready for her. It really gave us the special feeling that people really do care that we have a problem. We received this special treatment every place we went.

The rest of the day, we went where Stephanie wanted to go: the Jungle Cruise, the Mark Twain Riverboat, Pirates of the Caribbean, Bear Country Jamboree, the People Mover, the Autobahn, the King Arthur Carrousel, and Pinocchio's Journey.

The ride before us on the Carrousel had a live band riding the horses and playing instead of the piped-in music. Watching them play as they went around and around was neat.

Disneyland was very accommodating to us. We weren't required to wait in line, and they were ready to help with Stephanie and didn't make us feel awkward or hurried because we were slowing the line down. We all had a good time. We were all tired, but especially Stephanie.

Promise

Hebrews 13:5 (Living Bible)

Stay away from the love of money; be satisfied with what you have. For God has said, "I will never, *never* fail you nor forsake you."

Prayer

Dear Lord,

You know our financial needs even before we do. You know what this whole ordeal will end up costing us in lost wages, added expenses, etc. We have faith that You will provide for our needs.

Chapter 16

Memories Continue to be Made

As Stephanie continued to fight her battle with cancer and survived, we continued to make memories with her. Whenever she was physically able to and wanted to do something, we tried to do it. For instance, if she wanted to go to a movie or out to eat (She especially had cravings for Taco Bell's Mexican pizza), I stopped working and took her. That was where a lot of hidden expenses came in. I lost money by not working, and it cost money to get into the movies or to eat. And if I didn't take Roni with us, sometimes she felt left out. And she also needed to make memories with her sister. That was a hard situation but going into debt to help Stephanie and us go through this life-to-death process was worth the cost.

Stephanie knew she was dying, and she didn't seem to be bitter about it. She had accepted the fact and realized that we had done and were doing all we could to make it easier for her.

Her fifteenth birthday, March 10, 1989, was a wonderful example of how friends helped us make wonderful memories, as well as making their own. Anita Mendoza, her daughter Heather, and Laura Boynton, one of Stephanie's best friends, wanted to do something special for Stephanie.

This is how the day went.

I told Stephanie I would take her shopping with the money she had gotten in her birthday cards, but I wanted to get the car washed first. The car wash I wanted to use was way across town, and since we were "way across town" and close to her old school, Fairview Junior Academy, I said, "Why don't we stop at the school and you can say hi to all your friends?"

The school, of course, knew we were coming. The kids had made a banner and taped it in the front courtyard. Tables were set up with punch, cookies, chips and dip, and balloons. The banner said Happy Birthday Steph. They had drawn balloons on the banner and written in the balloons, "We love you" and "Happy 15th". The whole junior high came out for their lunch break and sang "Happy Birthday" to Stephanie and gave her a handful of cards. Two of her friends had gotten her two little stuffed animals.

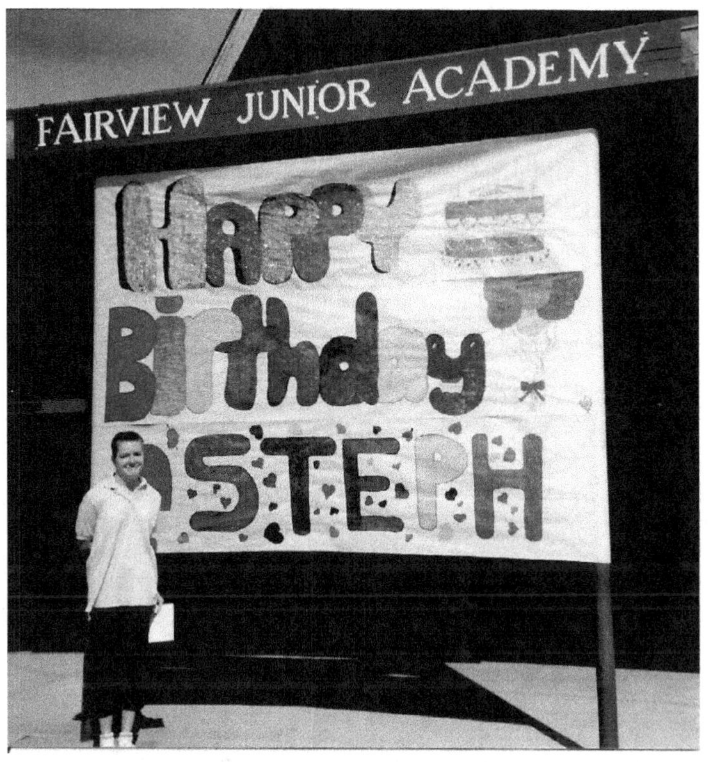

Then Anita, Heather, Laura, Roni, and I took Stephanie to a movie. It was a funny movie, so we were all laughing and feeling great. Then we went out to eat at Mimi's Café in Ontario, CA. We had told them it was Stephanie's birthday, so when they brought the dessert, they sang to her.

Afterward, we were home only fifteen minutes when the singing group that had sung to Stephanie in the hospital came to the door to see her. Anita had arranged for The Master's Plan to come sing about six songs for her. They even arranged their own version of "Happy Birthday to Stephanie."

Anita, Heather, and Laura had paid for this whole day. We all had a wonderful time. Stephanie's face was happy and surprised all day. When we went to the movie, she said, "Mom, we aren't going to be home in time for my tutor." So I had to tell her I had talked to him on Thursday and he knew about the whole day.

She went to bed very tired but very happy.

On April 6, 1989, Stephanie asked me if she had any say in what happened with her life-insurance money. So I asked her what she had in mind.

She said, "I would like for five thousand dollars to go to Roni for a new car and for you to have the rest to help pay some bills." She also said, "I don't want any slow, sad organ music at my funeral. I want it to be upbeat. Something like Amy Grant or the Goads. I am not sad that I am dying. I know you will miss me, but don't be sad for me."

I feel the need to explain Stephanie's life-insurance policy. Again, I feel God's guiding hands were at work. When Stephanie was one year old and Roni was five, I purchased a one-thousand-dollar life-insurance policy on each of them. Through the years, the agent would write or call about updating the policy. I told them I didn't care what they did as long as I didn't have to pay any more premium than I was. So when Stephanie was diagnosed with brain cancer, I called the company and asked what I actually had on the girls at that point. The agent called me back and said that, with all the updating and changes, I then had twenty-five thousand dollars on each girl.

If anyone reading has had to check on the cost of a funeral, you know that one thousand dollars will not cover the costs. I would like to give you a breakdown of what we found in our area for our closest cemetery and mortuary in 1989:

Cemetery plot	$650.00 or more
Cement bell (required by	$400.00
Interment & recording fee, opening & closing	$1,500.00
Headstone & installation fee	$900.00
Casket	$500.00 or more (we chose the next style up at $1,600.00
Total	$4,950.00

Now in 2018, it is closer to:

Cemetery plot	$9,300.00
Cement bell (required by law)	$1,390.00
Interment & recording fee, opening & closing	$1,500.00
Headstone & installation fee	$1,100.00
Processing fee & Sales tax	$260.00
Casket	$1,100.00 or more
Total	$14,650.00

I know most families don't have life insurance on their children. But I am so glad that God impressed me to purchase them when the girls were little. We didn't have five thousand dollars of extra cash on hand, and for the twenty-five to thirty dollars a year that we paid, we received twenty-five thousand dollars. Praise the Lord!

On April 15, 1989, the Goads put on a performance at a local church. They are a family that tours around, putting on Christian concerts and witnessing about the Lord. Steve and I heard them perform about a week before Stephanie was diagnosed with the tumor. They were very uplifting and gave us a lot of strength. We purchased about six of their tapes. When Stephanie was in the hospital, she listened to their tapes and would feel better. Stephanie, Steve, and I went to another of their concerts in October 1988.

Then we went again on that Saturday night in 1989. They sang and gave their testimonies, and they had an altar call. Stephanie wanted to go up, so Steve went with her. The sister, Carol Sue, came down and gave Stephanie a hug and prayed with her. The whole time Stephanie was getting hugged by Carol Sue, tears were streaming down my checks.

You know, crying can be very therapeutic. I felt as though it was cleansing my mind. It got rid of the little bit of anger and frustration creeping in.

They told Steve that a friend had told them about us, and they wanted to meet us and asked if we could wait after the service to see them. So we did. The family gathered around us and talked with us, prayed over us, and hugged us. They took our phone number and said they would call and check up on Stephanie. Stephanie was so happy but totally exhausted. When we got in the car to go home, Stephanie sat and just melted. She had no strength left. I asked her if she wanted me to belt her in, and all she could do was nod. So I belted her in and closed the door. When we got home, Steve had to carry her to bed because she was so tired she could not even walk. Even with her deterioration, I felt at peace. It was a wonderful experience.

Stephanie's courage and stamina witnessed to the Goads. They told us that they were starting to feel frustrated with their hectic tour of Europe and the United States, and they were starting to grumble, but after talking to Stephanie, they realized they had nothing to gripe about. They said that Stephanie's sweetness, gentleness, and lovingkindness really touched them and they would remember her always and especially in their prayers.

Stephanie Has Touched Me

by Anita Mendoza

I was given the honor one Sunday afternoon to sit with Stephanie. I was so excited about being asked. Stephanie's health was declining, and her speech was as soft as a summer breeze, whispering through her colorless lips. She was sitting in her favorite chair in the family room and watching her favorite movie, *Top Gun*. I sat down on the chair next to her and proceeded to read one of the beginning drafts of this book, which her mother was working on. As I finished reading the last words, Stephanie looked toward me with an immensely compassionate look. I looked up, tears in my eyes, my arms and legs weak. Then I stood up as she watched every move I was making.

I put the manuscript down and said, "Steph, you know God knew what He was doing when He chose your mom and dad."

So strong and proud with no questions or doubts, she looked at me and said, "I know."

Then I looked at her and said, "You are special too, you know."

She looked up at me and said, again just as strong and proud, "I know, and you are too."

Thank you, Steph, for sharing with me.

Promise

Psalms 23:1-6 (KJV)

The Lord is my shepherd; I shall not want. He maketh me to lie down in green pastures: he leadeth me beside the still waters. He restoreth my soul: he leadeth me in the paths of righteousness for his name's sake. Yea, though I walk through the valley of the shadow of death, I will fear no evil: for thou art with me; thy rod and thy staff they comfort me. Thou preparest a table before me in the presence of mine enemies: thou anointest my head with oil; my cup runneth over. Surely goodness and mercy shall follow me all the days of my life: and I will dwell in the house of the Lord forever.

Prayer

Dear Lord,

Thank you for being our shepherd. We are like lost sheep, unable to find our own way. Thank you for preparing the table before us.

Chapter 17

Stephanie's Last Days

On May 30, 1989, Stephanie was slowly getting worse. She was having frequent headaches and losing more and more control of her right side and some on her left side. That day, her blood pressure was so low that the hospice nurse couldn't even hear it, and her pulse was very erratic. Stephanie was becoming more restless. She rang her bell for something every fifteen minutes or so, and because her speech was becoming more and more affected, we were having a harder time figuring out what she needed. She was also starting to lose control of her bladder.

On June 6, 1989, when the hospice nurse came, Stephanie was really doing poorly. Her pulse was thready, and again the nurse couldn't get a blood pressure. Stephanie's color was very poor. The nurse didn't think Stephanie could last much longer. We called Pastor John, and he came over that evening and couldn't believe how bad Stephanie looked.

When he left, he told us, "I may not see her again."

When we told her goodnight, we didn't expect her to wake up in the morning. But she did wake up and looked better than she had for a long time.

Stephanie couldn't eat anymore—swallowing was too hard for her. She could down a couple sips of soda once in a while, but that was all.

Several people offered to stay with Stephanie. Some I knew wouldn't be able physically. They didn't realize how much care she took. Besides, we were reluctant to leave her. I suggested to people trying to help that they say, "I would like to come help you. Can I bring lunch and we sit and talk, or would you like to go out for lunch and let me stay with Stephanie?"

On July 14, 1989, Stephanie wanted to be held. I held her most of the morning and could feel her slowly going deeper and deeper into a coma. We couldn't rouse her at all the rest of the day.

On July 17, 1989, a Monday, the hospice nurse said Stephanie was showing all the signs of the final stages of life. She gave us a handout titled "Signs and Symptoms of approaching Death." We read it, and Stephanie had shown all of them:

1. Arms and legs may become cool to the touch, and the underside of the body may become darker in color. These symptoms are a result of blood circulation slowing down.

2. May spend more time sleeping and at times will be difficult to arouse. This is a result of a change in the body's metabolism.

3. May become increasingly confused about time, place, and identity of close and familiar people. Again, this is a result of body metabolism changes.

4. Incontinence (loss of control) of urine and bowel movements is often not a problem until death becomes imminent.

5. Oral secretions may become more profuse and collect in the back of the throat. You may have heard friends refer to a "death rattle." This symptom is a result of a decrease in the body's intake of fluids and inability to cough up normal saliva production.

6. Clarity of hearing and vision decrease slightly.

7. They may become restless, pulling at bed linen, and may have visions of people or things that you do not see. These symptoms are a result of a decrease in the oxygen circulating to the brain and a change in the body's metabolism.

8. They will have a decreased need for food and drink because the body will naturally begin to conserve energy, which is expended on these tasks.

9. During sleep, at first, you will notice breathing patterns change to an irregular pace where there may be ten-to-thirty-second periods of no breathing. These periods are referred to as "apnea." This symptom is very common and indicative of a decrease in circulation and buildup in the body's water products.

10. The amount of urine will decrease as death comes closer.

Because Stephanie was showing all these signs, we called all the relatives and closest friends, and they all came to spend some time with us and Stephanie and to help. That night, Marion, my stepmother, sat with Stephanie, holding her hand, rubbing her back, and talking to her. Her breathing just kept getting harder and harder.

On Wednesday afternoon, July 19, 1989, we thought it was all over. Stephanie turned blue and stayed that way for over half an hour. All of a sudden, she opened her eyes, her color came back better than it had been for weeks, and she pointed at her ceiling fan, wanting us to turn it off. She stayed semi alert all through Thursday.

In fact, Steve and two of Stephanie's best friends, Heather and Laura, washed Stephanie's hair. You could tell by Stephanie's face that she liked that and it felt good. We could not get her out of bed, so Steve was really ingenious. He turned her sideways in bed with her head just barely off the side. Then with a watering can and a bucket underneath, they washed her hair.

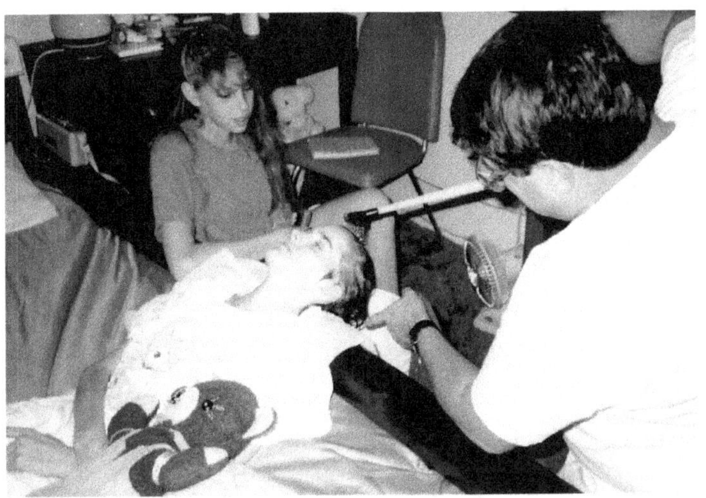

Marion stayed up with her again all Thursday night. She said Stephanie was awake and alert most of the night.

Friday, July 21, 1989, Stephanie was asleep and basically unmoving all day. Once in a while, she would squeeze our hands, but most of the time, she was in a really deep sleep. Saturday and Sunday, she slowly got worse. She was totally nonresponsive.

On Monday, July 24, 1989, I was home alone with Stephanie. Everyone had gone. I was trying to do some work on the computer because there was nothing I could do for Stephanie. I was very nervous, frustrated, anxious, and anything else you could think of, and I needed to do something, so I worked. I checked Stephanie every ten minutes. She was breathing so hard that her whole body was working just to breathe.

Every time I looked at her, I cried and prayed that she would die and be out of the struggle, that she could rest in peace. At twenty till one in the afternoon, I kneeled by her and held her and told her that it was okay to stop fighting, that it was okay to rest and go to sleep in Jesus. Ten minutes later, I went in and at once knew she was at peace. Stephanie had died with her bear Jason in her arms.

I just lay down beside her and held her for five minutes. Then I got up and called hospice, Pastor Lenart, Pastor Bottroff, Anita Mendoza, and Fuji Medical Systems to get hold of Steve. My dad was already on his way from Oxnard and was due any minute. Before anyone got there, I got out the handout that hospice had given us and read the section titled "How Would You Know Death Has Occurred?"

1. No breathing
2. No heartbeat
3. Loss of control of bowel and bladder
4. Eyelids slightly open
5. Eyes fixed on a certain spot
6. Jaw relaxed and mouth slightly open

Anita and my Dad pulled up at the same time. Ten minutes later, Pastor Bottroff showed up. About five minutes after that, the hospice nurse came. Right after that, the mortician came, and about five minutes after that, Steve got home.

Once everyone arrived, I felt at a loss, waiting for everyone to tell me what to do. Everything was happening so quickly. The mortician told us when Stephanie would be ready for the visitation and when the funeral parlor would be available, Pastor Bottroff made sure the church would be available for the funeral, and within forty-five minutes, Anita and my sister, LaVon, were calling everyone with all the details. Stephanie had died Monday afternoon, the visitation would be Wednesday night, and the funeral would be Thursday morning, with a potluck lunch afterward.

As the morticians were taking Stephanie away, I handed them Jason and asked that it be buried with her. He had been through everything with her. He had been her support. She had died with him in her arms, and he would stay there.

After everyone left that night, I just had a sense of relief. It was over. It was over for Stephanie—no more pain, no more frustration over not being able to do what she used to do, no more struggling just to breathe. It was also over for me. I was not tied down any more. I did not have to lift her and change her diaper. I didn't have to stay home all the time. You know, I really didn't feel guilty about my feelings of relief. In fact, I think I was more surprised than anything else. I had never been resentful about having to stay home a lot and take care of Stephanie, so I guess that is why I didn't feel guilty about feeling relieved.

Am I Ready?

by Grampa

As I think back over the period of Stephanie's two years of terminal illness, my most prominent impression, aside from the initial shock and continuing grief, was Stephanie's own reaction and attitude. Her strong faith and acceptance of her condition and its expected outcome were an inspiration to me. I saw every indication that she had placed herself in the hands of the Lord and was looking beyond the immediate future to a peaceful and joyous life in His eternal kingdom of love. She was ready! And more than that, her first concern was for her family. Would I be that ready? I hope so and like to think so.

One small episode I recall, which I think illustrates her attitude, took place in the later stages of her illness. She was in bed and couldn't move much or talk. I stepped into her room and spoke to her, identifying myself as Grandpa, and she looked at me and responded by wiggling her fingers at me in acknowledgement and greeting. She seemed to be saying, "I love you."

Promise

John 14:1-3 (KJV)

Let not your heart be troubled: ye believe in God, believe also in me. In my Father's house are many mansions: if it were not so, I would have told you. I go to prepare a place for you. And if I go and prepare a place for you, I will come again, and receive you unto myself; that where I am, there ye may be also.

Prayer

Dear Lord,

Thank you for coming to earth and dying for us. Thank you for preparing a place for us in heaven to be with you. We cannot wait for your second return so that we may all be together again.

Chapter 18

Farewell

The following Tuesday, I went through all our family picture albums and pulled out the best of Stephanie and any that had her with special friends and relatives. I made up a separate album, which took me all day because I sat there looking at each picture and remembering all the wonderful times we'd had. It hurt, and I cried, but It felt good. It made me realize that we had done a lot as a family. I don't think we could have done much more in just fifteen years. I took this special "Stephanie album" to the funeral parlor for the visitation, and all the people loved it, especially if they found pictures of themselves with Stephanie.

While I was making this album, Steve was making a special audio tape to be played at the funeral before and after the service because Stephanie had said what she did and did not want. When Steve finished the tape, he played it back, but it had not recorded evenly, and he was very unhappy, but emotionally he couldn't handle redoing it just then, so he said he would remake it on Thursday morning. Therefore, while

Grandma and Grandpa Squier and I went to the church Thursday morning to put paper tablecloths on the lunch tables, Steve redid the tape after saying a prayer for God to lead him as to what songs to include. It came out perfect. We heard several people comment after the funeral how wonderful the music was. One person said she was holding her emotions okay until, as she was walking down the aisle to go past Stephanie, someone on the tape started singing the simple children's song, "Jesus Loves Me." You know, there were over three hundred people at Stephanie's funeral, and we have no idea how many people were affected by either the picture album or the music. All we know is that for Steve and me, they were major parts of our saying good-bye to Stephanie.

As we were planning the final touches for Stephanie's funeral, we were impressed with how important it was as a witness of God's great love. We'd felt God leading in the making of the picture album and the music tape. We also told the pastors we wanted them to talk briefly about our belief in the state of the dead and not make a major sermon out of it. When we asked The Master's Plan to sing, they asked what songs we wanted, and we just said for them to pray about it and sing whatever God impressed them to sing.

You know, when we let God lead, He does a wonderful job. Everything fell into place, and it was a wonderful service.

The church we were in was not set up so that the family was out of sight. We had to sit on the front row. What we did not plan was that at the end of the service, when everyone came down past the casket, they walked right past us.

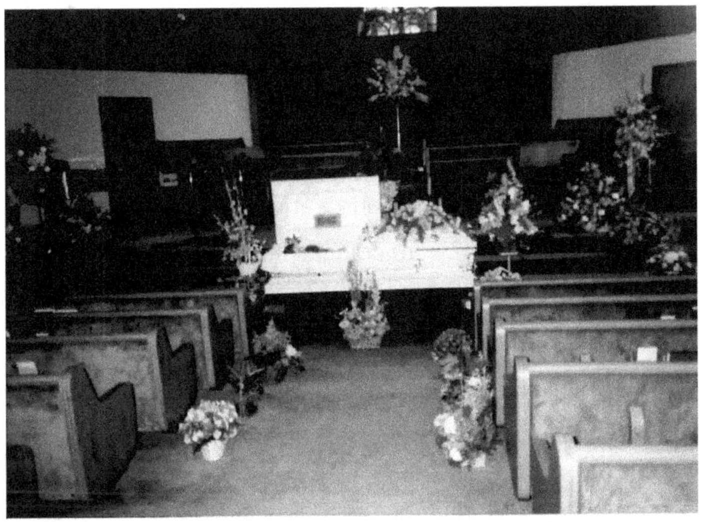

The first person down was a good friend, and they hugged Steve and me. My first reaction was "Oh no! I won't be able to handle everyone hugging me." But it was wonderful. I think that should be the tradition. Partway through, it dawned on me that God was giving me hugs through all these people. The power of touch is amazing. We were tired, but we felt a lot better. I was amazed by the thought that over three hundred people were there, but that was just a fraction of the people that Stephanie's life had touched.

For a couple years, people would come up to us and say how wonderful that service was. They told us how they were all down and depressed when they came because the life of a fifteen-year-old was over. But they left at peace and not depressed anymore. Stephanie is resting in peace, asleep till

Jesus's second coming, when He comes to take us all to heaven for eternity. Just think, Stephanie will be fifteen years old when we get to heaven, and I'll get to raise her in a perfect world with Jesus right there helping me. What a privilege and an honor.

I was told on October 7, 1989, that Heather and Laura had gone to Stephanie's grave and sat on the grass and talked about everything they were doing at school and about all their friends. They had taken balloons and flowers. They wrote messages to Stephanie on the balloons, and after about half an hour, they let the balloons go, and just as they did, a breeze came up, but her balloons caught a thermal draft and went straight up out of sight. When Laura's grandma told me this, I cried tears of joy. It is good for a mother to hear about how her child has affected people for the good.

Yes, I miss Stephanie, and I expect I will always miss her. After all, she was one of the major parts of my life. She was part of me. I would like to quote from a book I'VE been reading.

Turn Your Hurts into Healing

by V. Gilbert Beers

I have heard that time heals wounds, but I do not believe that is true. Time covers wounds, applies a Band-Aid over them, perhaps even a thin scab over them. They become less visible. But the wounds remain. What we have is not a scar, symbol of healing, but bleeding wounds, if not bleeding externally, bleeding internally.

If you are still grieving for the loss of someone important to you and wonder why, be assured you are a member of the Fellowship of the Wounded. You, like I, will always be wounded. Skin heals but hearts do not... I believe my wife and I will always be wounded because we will always bleed for our son. If we heal completely it suggests we are over it, and I honestly hope that I never reach the point where I am over it, because then I will no longer miss him, no longer grieve for him, no longer pay tribute to him and what he brought into our lives. No, we really do not want to get over it. but we do want to be changed people. Whole people again. Our wholeness does not embrace a living son, as it once did, but memories of a living son. It embraces a desire to make our son's life worthwhile, redemptive... for those of you who mourn, do not shrink from true mourning. You may indeed be fortunate, not because you have something to cause you to mourn, but because in your suffering you will encounter comfort. I think what Jesus is telling us is this: when you have suffered loss, mourn! Don't hold back. Someone said that we must bury our dead (or those lost in some other way) or we will carry them like an albatross throughout our lifetimes. In other words, if you refuse to mourn you will always carry that burden that mourning could have removed from you. I think that is what Jesus is saying. Mourning removes the burden that loss placed upon you. Comfort is the relief you enjoy when that burden is lifted. Could we rephrase Matthew 5:4, "those who mourn are fortunate, for they shall discover the relief of having their burden of loss lifted." The loss is not lifted, but the burden imposed by that loss is.

That is how we feel about Stephanie. That is why we have gone through the extremely painful process of writing this book. We feel that if one person can be helped, it is worth it.

I would like to quote one more paragraph, this time from *Washington!*, a book in the Wagons West series, by Dana Fuller Ross: "There is nothing harder to accept then the finality of death, but we've got to accept it because we have no real choice. It may be cruel, and it may be senseless, but we do no favors for the dead by overindulging our grief for them, and we must keep in mind that life is to be lived by and for the living."

Once more from *Turn Your Hurts into Healing*, by V. Gilbert Beers: "Team up with God in making your hurts for something, and thus participate in His great plan of redemption."

On April 25, 1990, we received a letter from one of the teachers at Fairview Junior Academy.

> Dear Mr. and Mrs. Leber,   4-18-90
>
> Dawn Brehms sent me a poem she wrote about Stephanie and requested I send it to you — she is a very sensitive girl and expresses herself well... hope you enjoy it!
>
> Dana Tiller

She sent us a copy of a poem written by Dawn Brehms to Stephanie. She was a classmate of Stephanie's.

Sleeping in Christ

Here you lay
asleep in Christ
It seems like
years
Since the last
of each other we
have seen.
But only yesterday
you were alive + well.

Here you lay.
asleep in Christ.
waiting for resurrection
day.
like morning dew.
awaiting the dawning
of the sun.

My dear friend
you a warning
for when Christ
        says

Arise! Arise!
you will come forth
a new & glorious
        being

Sleep peacfful
    · My dear
        beutiful
        friend.

        Dawn
        Brehm
        — 1990 —

On May 12, 1990, the day before Mother's Day, our church was having a special prayer for mothers. As others were going down to kneel and have special prayer, a friend's four-year-old daughter came over to me, sat in my lap, and whispered, "Stephanie's not here, but you will be with her again in heaven." Then she gave me a big hug. Yes, I cried, but it was a good cry. I was happy that someone cared and remembered. I hope memories like these continue forever.

Footprints

One night a man had a dream. He dreamed he was walking along the beach with the Lord. Across the sky flashed scenes from his life. For each scene, he noticed two sets of footprints in the sand: one belonging to him, the other to the Lord. When the last scene of his life flashed before him, he looked back at the footprints in the sand. He noticed that many times along the path of his life there was only one set of footprints. He also noticed that it happened at the very lowest and saddest times of his life.

This really bothered him and he questioned the Lord about it. "Lord, You said that once I decided to follow You, You'd walk with me all the way. But I have noticed that during the most troublesome times in my life, there is only one set of footprints. I don't understand why when I needed You most You would leave me."

The Lord replied, "My son, My precious child, I love you and would never leave you. During your times of trial and suffering, when you see only one set of footprints, it was then that I carried you."

Author Unknown

Extra Pictures

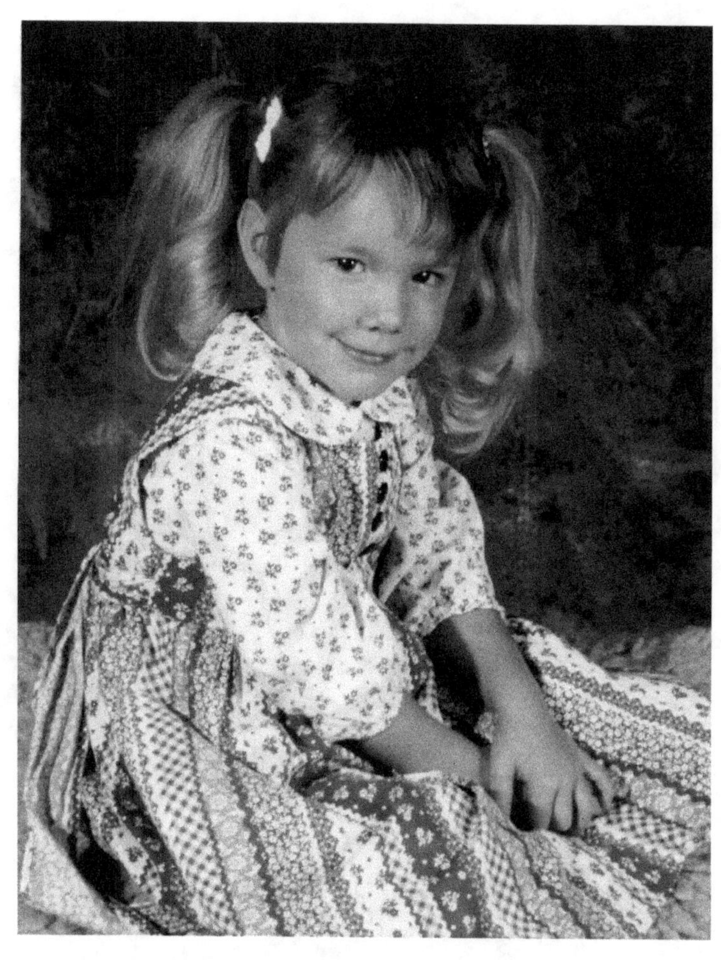

Mom's Favorite Picture

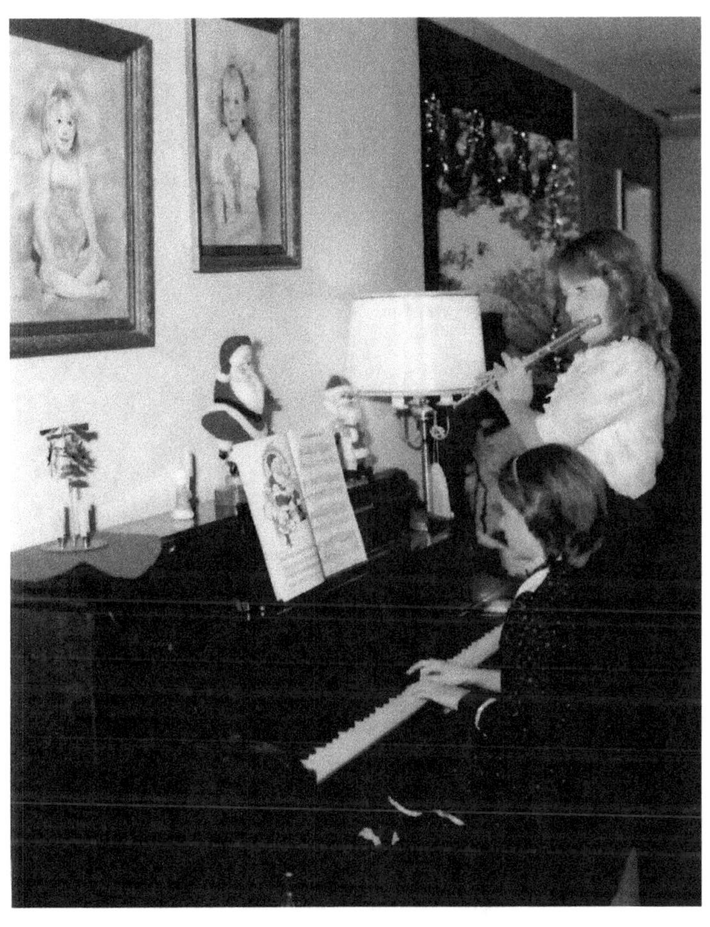

Stephie and Roni Playing Music for Christmas

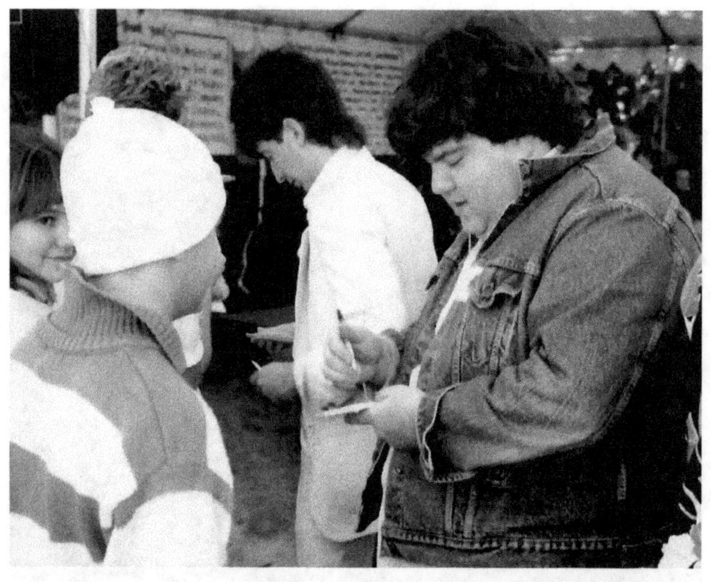

Stephanie Getting Autographs from Dan Schneider & Dan Frishman (from *Head of the Class*) at Ronald McDonald's Cancer Event in Hollywood

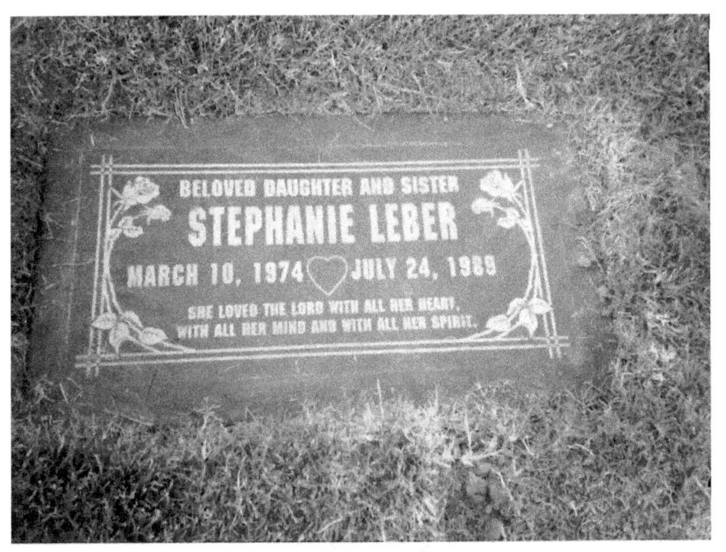

Stephanie Ellen Leber

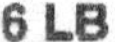

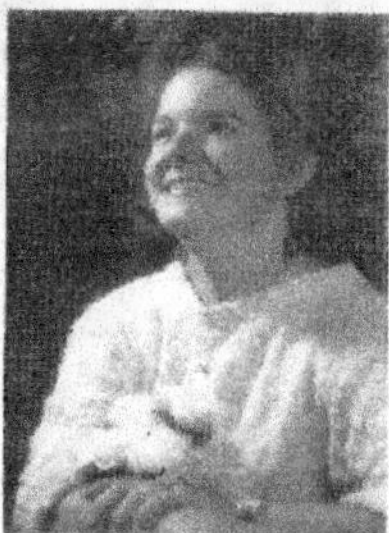

The American Cancer Society put pictures of people who had died of cancer on bags then had school children color the back of each bag.

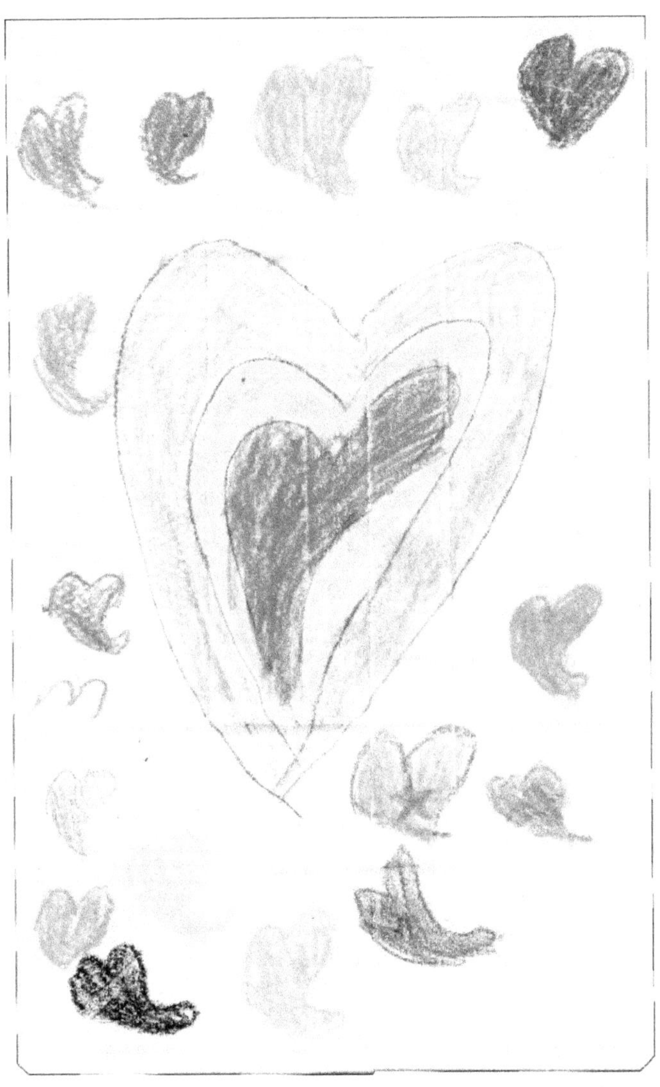

The American Cancer Society put on a 24-hour cancer walk at a local school track. They lined the track with bags with candles in them.

EPILOGUE

I wrote this book during the time of Stephanie's illness. Writing it helped me to keep things in perspective while processing everything that was happening to our family. Getting my feeling out somehow, while not burdening other people, was very therapeutic for me.

At first, I think I started writing simply in order to keep a journal for the questions that the doctors were asking me. I needed to keep a timeline of events and progressing symptoms in Stephanie's life, beginning with the headache. Thus, I would record when she had them and how severe they were, etc.

Eventually, other people started to ask me to write more about the details of Stephanie's life because she seemed so accepting of her condition, and that was unexpected for many people. They wanted to know more about her, curious about where that sense of peace came from.

After the manuscript was complete, I did send it off to several publishers, but nobody wanted to publish it at that time. None of the companies ever gave a reason, so for many years, I never knew what they thought of it. Maybe I'll never know.

Years passed, and the manuscript sat in a drawer somewhere.

Then, not too many months back, a friend and I found the story as we were going through some papers after my husband died. The friend wanted to know what it was about, so I told him about this story about Stephanie, which no publishers wanted to handle. Well, he started bugging me to get the manuscript edited and told me that self-publishing was much more common and easier than it had ever been, so I finally gave in and agreed.

You're holding the results of this literary resurrection in your hands now.

Appendix I

Chronology of Major Events and Developments

February 1974

- ♥ Steve baptized as SDA

March 10, 1974

- ♥ Stephanie born

1983 – 1987

- ♥ Migraine headaches

October 20, 1987

- ♥ Migraine headaches more frequent
- ♥ Other physical symptoms
- ♥ CT and MRI scans revealed brain tumor
- ♥ Roni home from SPA

November 4, 1987

- ♥ Angio in morning
- ♥ Entire body of school students visit Stephanie at hospital in four school buses
- ♥ Evening: anointing service

November 5, 1987

- ♥ Initial surgery

November 6, 1987

- ♥ Emergency burr-hole surgery

November 7, 1987

- ♥ Traumatic: head bandaged, drain tubes,
- ♥ Intravenous injections, catheter

- ♥ Respirator

November 12, 1987

- ♥ Third surgery: shunt instead of drain tube

November 13, 1987

- ♥ Removed respirator—speech difficulty

November 19, 1987

- ♥ Home two weeks after initial surgery

December 4-19, 1987

- ♥ Hawaii

December 17 to February 10, 1988

- ♥ Radiation treatments

February 11-15, 1988

- ♥ Losing coordination, lethargic

February 17, 1988

- ♥ CT scan: tumor appeared much larger
- ♥ Decided against further surgery
- ♥ Stephanie sent home

February 21, 1988

- ♥ Open house for Stephanie

March 17, 1988

- ♥ MRI showed cyst with fluid

March 18, 1988

- ♥ Stephanie to hospital

March 19, 1988

- ♥ Fourth surgery: removed fluid from cyst

March 23, 1988

- ♥ Stephanie sent home

April 4 to June 1988

♥ Stephanie occasionally attended school

May 8, 1988

♥ Headache & vomiting-CT scan negative

♥ Flu or upset stomach?

June 9, 1988

♥ Stephanie graduated from eighth grade

September 1988

♥ Tried school but managed only two days in two weeks

♥ Home tutoring started again

October 19, 1988

♥ MRI scan showed no live tissue in tumor: "Miracle!"

January 21-24, 1989

♥ Headaches and vomiting

♥ Right side "weird": arm, leg, and face

January 24, 1989

♥ MRI showed tumor alive and growing

January 25, 1989

♥ Stephanie to hospital

January 26, 1989

♥ Fifth surgery: additional shunt

January 28, 1989

♥ Stephanie sent home

February 16, 1989

♥ No more doctors could do

March 8, 1989

♥   Disneyland

March 10, 1989

♥   Stephanie's birthday

April 15, 1989

♥   The Goads concert

July 24, 1989

♥   Death

July 27, 1989

♥   Funeral

Appendix II

Supportive Community Organizations

Several organizations are available to help families with children with any form of cancer or terminal illness. Here are the ones that have helped us:

1. Starlight Foundation, (310) 479-1212
2. Camp Ronald McDonald for Good Times, 56400 Apple Canyon Road, Mountain Center, CA 92561; (951) 659-4609
3. Candlelighters Childhood Cancer Foundation of the Inland Empire, 11155 Mountain View Ave. #105, Loma Linda, CA 92354; (909) 558-3419
4. Hospice, usually available through your local hospital.

A lot of other foundations exist, but these are the ones that have helped us.

If you need financial assistance, you may qualify for help from the Department of Public Health, California Children Services, at 351 N. Mountain View Avenue, San Bernardino, CA 92415-0010. Phone: (909) 387-6200.

9 781727 149890